AF866957

The Practice of Clinical Governance

Luis Prado • Sidney Chandrasiri

The Practice of Clinical Governance

A Practical Guide for Healthcare Leaders

Springer

Luis Prado
Australian Institute of Health Executives (AIHE)
Brisbane, QLD, Australia

Royal Australasian College of Medical Administrators (RACMA)
Melbourne, VIC, Australia

Sidney Chandrasiri
Australian Institute of Health Executives (AIHE)
Brisbane, QLD, Australia

Royal Australasian College of Medical Administrators (RACMA)
Melbourne, VIC, Australia

ISBN 978-981-19-7895-1 ISBN 978-981-19-7896-8 (eBook)
https://doi.org/10.1007/978-981-19-7896-8

© The Editor(s) (if applicable) and The Author(s), under exclusive license to Springer Nature Singapore Pte Ltd. 2026

This work is subject to copyright. All rights are solely and exclusively licensed by the Publisher, whether the whole or part of the material is concerned, specifically the rights of translation, reprinting, reuse of illustrations, recitation, broadcasting, reproduction on microfilms or in any other physical way, and transmission or information storage and retrieval, electronic adaptation, computer software, or by similar or dissimilar methodology now known or hereafter developed.
The use of general descriptive names, registered names, trademarks, service marks, etc. in this publication does not imply, even in the absence of a specific statement, that such names are exempt from the relevant protective laws and regulations and therefore free for general use.
The publisher, the authors and the editors are safe to assume that the advice and information in this book are believed to be true and accurate at the date of publication. Neither the publisher nor the authors or the editors give a warranty, expressed or implied, with respect to the material contained herein or for any errors or omissions that may have been made. The publisher remains neutral with regard to jurisdictional claims in published maps and institutional affiliations.

This Springer imprint is published by the registered company Springer Nature Singapore Pte Ltd.
The registered company address is: 152 Beach Road, #21-01/04 Gateway East, Singapore 189721, Singapore

If disposing of this product, please recycle the paper.

Disclaimer

The Case studies including clinical cases used in this book are fictional and have no relationship to any person living or dead or any organisations and any resemblance to any individuals or organisations is coincidental.

Contents

About the Authors

Luis Prado, MBBS FRACGP FCHSM FACHE FRACMA FACMQ GAICD is a Medical Graduate of the University of Queensland, Fellow of the Royal Australasian College of Medical Administrators, Fellow of the Royal Australian College of General Practitioners, Fellow of the American College of Healthcare Executives, Fellow of the American College of Medical Quality, Fellow of the Australasian College of Health Service Management, and Graduate of the Australian Institute of Company Directors. He has held several senior Healthcare and Medical Executive leadership roles across both the public and private healthcare sectors in Australia, along with key Board Director roles in the for-profit and not-for profit sectors. He is leading national expert in clinical governance presenting multiple papers both in Australia and Internationally.

He is an Affiliate Professor at the Deakin University School of Medicine, Adjunct Professor at the Queensland University of Technology School of Medicine, and Adjunct Associate Professor of the University of Queensland Medical School has been actively involved in leading medical education and research across private and public healthcare organisations and specialty medical colleges. He is the Chief Academic Officer of the Australian Institute of Health Executives (AIHE).

Sidney Chandrasiri, MBBS FRACMA FCHSM MHM GAICD is a Medical Graduate of the University of New South Wales, Fellow of the Royal Australasian College of Medical Administrators, Fellow of the Australasian College of Health Service Management, Graduate of the Australian Institute of Company Directors, holds a master's in Health Management and Certification in Health Informatics and is a graduate of the highly selective Harvard Business School Intensive Program on Value Based Healthcare.

She has held a number of Health Executive and Medical Leadership roles across the private and public healthcare sectors in both metropolitan and regional settings across five states in Australia, including Board Director roles in community health and hospital health service boards. She has been a sentinel event reviewer for the Victorian Department of Health, has lectured on health system management to postgraduate students and medical administration trainees, is a speaker at multiple medical forums across Australia, and publishes widely in the field of medical leadership. Her portfolio encompasses executive health service leadership, clinical services design, strategic planning, medical workforce strategy and numerous areas across clinical governance and hospital operations in public and private health services. In addition Dr Chandrasiri is the Chief Executive of the Australian Institute of Health Executives (AIHE) and Chair of the AIHE Charitable Foundation.

1 Clinical Governance: An Overview

Clinical governance is a notion that is core to the management and leadership of health services. In its simplest form, it is a system of checks and balances that helps ensure health services are governed and operated in a safe and effective manner, with continued improvement in the delivery of high-quality patient care. It provides a framework for the prioritisation of decisions and actions based on their impact on patient safety. Clinical governance comprises the combination of several constituent parts: systems, processes, leadership, and staff, with clear accountability for providing safe, effective, appropriate, and patient-centred care, built on an organisational culture of continuous quality improvement (Fig. 1.1).

The purpose of clinical governance is to ensure that high quality care is being delivered to the right patient, on time, and in a coordinated way. It is, in effect, a system that governs the design and delivery of safe and effective clinical care. Clinical governance is realised through a range of strategies and actions that are commonly outlined in an overarching clinical governance framework. These include the development of organisational structures and processes to ensure a number of

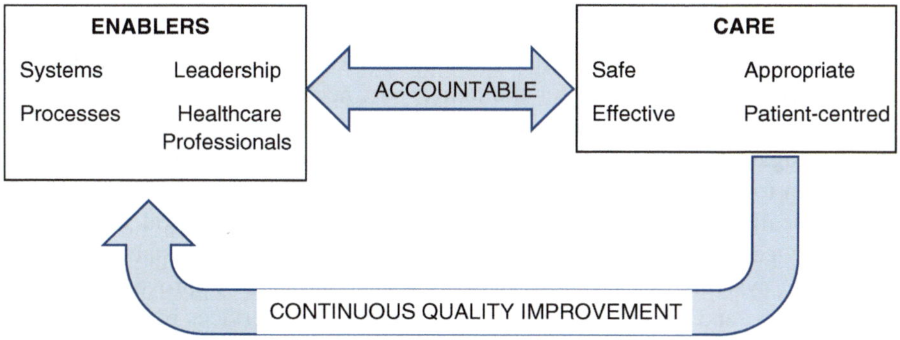

Fig. 1.1 Components of clinical governance

© The Author(s), under exclusive license to Springer Nature Singapore Pte Ltd. 2026
L. Prado, S. Chandrasiri, *The Practice of Clinical Governance*,
https://doi.org/10.1007/978-981-19-7896-8_1

key outcomes, including clear accountability, quality assurance, continuous improvement, clinical and operational effectiveness, adherence to evidence-based clinical practice, the identification and appropriate management of clinical incidents, and the proactive mitigation of risk where it exists.

From a practical standpoint, adopting a perspective of 'leading via clinical governance' is key to successfully meeting the multiple challenges that healthcare leaders are confronted with. Adopting such a mindset ensures that patient safety is at the forefront of all decision-making and fosters a degree of both collective and individual accountability in ensuring the best possible outcomes for patients.

There are five key elements that underpin a good clinical governance system. These define the areas in which appropriate systems and processes need to be established:

- Strong, authentic, and effective leadership at the level of the Health Service Board, Executive, and the frontline, is critical in setting the tone and standard of clinical governance across an organisation.
- The development of an organisation-wide clinical governance framework or strategy, with endorsement and commitment to its implementation by the leadership.
- Undertaking continuous benchmarking with external health services and national/international quality standards and evaluating the safety culture of an organisation helps demonstrate this commitment and engages front-line staff in clinical governance activities.
- An organisational culture where clinical governance, quality, and safety are entrenched and embedded. Health care leaders need to establish systems where quality and safety risks are actively monitored, incidents are readily identified, communicated, and appropriately responded to, and learnings and recommendations arising from these are disseminated throughout the organisation to prevent recurrence.
- Ensuring an understanding of and a commitment to accountability for clinical governance at the various governance levels of an organisation.

The role of *Health Service Boards* in clinical governance is to provide leadership, direction, and oversight for the delivery of healthcare services within their jurisdiction. This includes setting standards for the quality of care, monitoring performance against those standards, and taking action to address any areas of concern. In addition to operational and fiscal oversight, Board Directors of health services are specifically held accountable for the safety and quality of clinical services the health service provides and the extent to which they oversee the establishment of appropriate systems that are designed to ensure continuous improvement in the safety, quality, and effective clinical risk management of services being delivered. This includes the responsibility for setting expectations at all levels of the health service regarding the standard of clinical governance that is acceptable to the Board, empowering and enabling executive teams to create and promote positive safety culture, and driving performance improvement through measurement, review, and benchmarking activities.

In Australia, as in most health systems, legislation and regulation stipulates that Boards of metropolitan and regional/rural health services ensure systems are in place to monitor and improve the quality and effectiveness of health services and to identify and respond to any deficiencies or gaps identified.

The *Chief Executive (CE) and Executive management team* of a health service are responsible for setting the overall direction and strategy of the organisation. In the context of clinical governance, the Chief Executive, Chief Medical Officer (CMO), Chief Nursing Officer (CNO), or similar roles that make up the Clinical Executive (depending on the size, structure, and complexity of the organisation) have several key responsibilities in this regard. These include:

1. *Providing leadership*: The CE and CMO/CNO set the tone for the organisation and hold responsibility for ensuring that the organisation is committed to delivering high-quality care. They should provide clear guidance and support to staff to help them understand the importance of clinical governance and the role that each member of their staff plays in delivering safe, effective, and high-quality care.
2. *Ensuring compliance*: The CE and CMO/CNO are responsible for ensuring that the organisation is compliant with all relevant laws, regulations, and standards. This includes ensuring that appropriate policies and procedures are in place to support patient safety and confidentiality and that the organisation meets its obligations under relevant legislation and accreditation standards.
3. *Overseeing risk management*: The CE and CMO/CNO are responsible for overseeing the organisation's risk management strategies and for ensuring that appropriate measures are put in place to mitigate any risks to patients and staff.
4. *Promoting continuous improvement*: The CE and CMO/CNO should promote a culture of continuous improvement within the organisation, encouraging staff to embrace change and to continuously look for ways to improve the quality of care they provide.
5. *Supporting clinical governance committees*: The CE and CMO/CNO should support the work of clinical governance committees, providing them with the resources and support they need to effectively fulfil their role in ensuring the quality of care.

1.1 Patient-Centredness in Clinical Governance

Patient-centred clinical governance is a simple, yet highly effective approach to clinical governance that places the needs and perspectives of patients at the centre of all decision-making and designing of processes. In a patient-centred clinical governance system, the focus is placed on improving the quality and safety of care in a way that is tailored to the individual needs and preferences of the patient. It promotes encouraging patients to actively participate in their own care, to providing feedback on the quality of care they receive, and to informing continuous improvement of the clinical governance system of the organisation. The requirement for ensuring active involvement of patients in their care decisions, as well as for facilitating the participation of and advocacy for patients in the workings of clinical governance committees and activities, is enshrined in the *Australian National Safety and Quality Health Service (NSQHS) Standards*. Adhering to ongoing hospital accreditation requirements against key national standards, such as the *Partnering with Consumers (NSQHS) standard* means that patient safety remains a top priority, that processes and procedures are in place to minimise the risk of harm to patients, and that patients are seen as partners in the planning, design, delivery, measurement, and evaluation of the clinical services and governance systems of an organisation.

The monitoring and evaluation of patient-reported outcome measures (PROMs) and patient-reported experience measures (PREMs) are further mechanisms by which clinical governance systems and processes can be continuously informed by, and modified for, the direct improvement of patient care as a result.

Informed patient consent including informed financial consent is a key component of ensuring patient-centred clinical governance, in which the patient is provided with all relevant information they need to make an informed decision about their medical treatment or care. The goal of informed patient consent is to ensure that patients have the information they need to understand the risks and benefits of a proposed treatment or procedure and to make an informed decision on whether they should proceed with the recommended treatment or procedure. Key elements of informed patient consent include the provision of clear, concise, and easy-to-understand information about their medical condition, treatment/procedure, and any risks and benefits, in addition to engaging in a discussion with the patient to clarify any questions or concerns. Informed consent requires that patients are free to make a voluntary choice about their medical treatments and are not subjected to coercion or undue influence, and it ensures that patients are aware of their right to withdraw this consent at any time. Informed patient consent is an important aspect of patient-centred care, where health services can promote patient autonomy and choice, and can build their trust and confidence in the health system.

Ensuring transparent, honest, and *continuous open disclosure* with patients and families in the event of adverse events is another example of how trust and confidence in the organisation can be maintained or strengthened at times of difficulty. To facilitate and integrate this practice of patient-centred clinical governance into the fabric of an organisation, most hospitals establish structures such as patient advocacy committees, create patient ambassador roles, or enable access to community consumer partnerships.

1.2 Effective Clinical Practice

Fundamental to good clinical governance is the provision of good clinical care. Every clinician has a role in keeping patients safe and providing a good patient experience. Providing clinicians access to evidence-based best practices in their relevant specialities and clinical fields, clinical decision support tools such as clinical databases, up-to-date clinical care resources and guidelines, protocols, and care pathways are examples demonstrative of facilitating a high standard of clinical practice. Encouraging interdisciplinary collaboration and peer discussion among healthcare providers ensures that patients receive coordinated and effective care and reduces the risk of harm. Mutidisciplinary reviews, mortality and morbidity meetings, incident review processes, case conferences, clinical escalation procedures, and clinical handover standards are further mechanisms that allow for constructive peer review and professional discussion in the continuous improvement of clinical practice.

Evaluation of clinical outcomes via clinical audits, and benchmarking these against internal and external clinical registries and peer health services, facilitates the early identification of any unwarranted clinical practice variations. Setting up systems for the safe introduction of new technologies, clinical innovations, translational research, and outcome-based clinical trials further ensures contemporaneous and effective clinical practice is entrenched within a clinical governance framework.

1.3 Effective Clinical Workforce

An effective clinical workforce refers to a team of healthcare professionals who have the necessary knowledge, skills, experience, and resources to provide high-quality care to patients. An effective clinical workforce is essential for ensuring the delivery of safe, effective, appropriate, and patient-centred care.

Credentialing and defining the scope of practice are two important processes in healthcare that help to ensure clinicians have the necessary skills, knowledge, and experience to deliver safe and effective care to patients. Credentialing is the process of verifying the qualifications and competence of clinicians to ensure they have the appropriate education, training, and experience to provide the relevant care to patients. Defining the scope of practice refers to the process of determining the specific tasks, procedures, and responsibilities that a clinician is qualified and authorised to perform. The scope of practice is determined by their education, training, and experience as well as by the clinical capability and resource availability at the hospital site where they are delivering care.

From an organisational perspective, *workforce planning* ensures that the clinical workforce has the right mix of skills and experience to meet the needs of the patient cohort it serves.

Providing *professional development* opportunities to clinicians helps them stay up to date with the latest clinical practices and technologies, and ensuring that appropriate *clinical supervision* and support is provided to clinicians assures an effective clinical workforce for the delivery of safe, high-quality care.

1.4 Risk Management

The complexity of healthcare dictates that a key role of the healthcare leader is the management and mitigation of inherent risks within their domains. Managing risk from a clinical governance perspective involves identifying and managing risks that exist across clinical and patient safety, financial, operational, and other enterprise risks. It includes ensuring there are systems set up to identify and document organisational risk in risk registers, using clinical and operational data collected by the health service. This data is used in the continuous assessment of risk severity and likelihood, and to regularly report these to the governing body, doctors, and staff.

Risk management systems used in healthcare organisations must also include strategies, actions and clear role accountabilities for mitigating the risks that have been identified. Similarly, incident management systems play a critical role in recording and monitoring incidents and are used in identifying clinical and non-clinical risks in both private and public health services. It is prudent to periodically monitor the health service's performance in relation to the management of risks at all governing levels of the organisation, including conducting internal and external audits on the design and performance of these systems. Components that are crucial in setting up and maintaining an effective risk management system at a health service include establishing risk registers, incident management systems, policies and procedures to inform practice, tools to audit policy and practice, and processes to ensure legislative/regulatory compliance. Ensuring appropriate medico-legal review of clinical incidents, including the reporting of 'sentinel events' and implementing findings resulting from coronial and similar processes, will comprise a key part of a risk management system.

1.5 Organisational Culture

Implementing improvements or changes to clinical governance systems and managing cultural shifts within organisations requires careful leveraging of the above elements. Using meaningful benchmarks, quality, and clinical data to inform evidence-based practice in both the clinical and administrative spheres, and ensuring a patient-centred approach, will position healthcare leaders to effectively engage, communicate, and facilitate a whole-of-hospital approach to clinical governance. Executive commitment and Board endorsement are crucial in setting the tone and standard of clinical governance at an organisation. Sponsoring 'clinical champions' to advocate for and lead clinical governance improvement at the front line requires having specific education and training programs to ensure staff and doctors receive training in clinical governance.

A '*dyad management structure*' where clinicians and management work in close partnership to achieve a desired culture shift and/or improvement in clinical governance, will yield the most effective outcomes. The healthcare leader must be aware and be willing to navigate the resistance that they will no doubt face in attempting cultural change to embed clinical governance practices. The impact of long-standing legacy systems, 'widely-held' beliefs, and defensive posturing that will be encountered will be directly dependent on and instrumental in having precipitated the inherent culture of an organisation. Research shows that organisations with strong dyad leadership teams are better equipped to successfully manage the clinical and operational complexities of healthcare.

The *triad leadership model*, characterised by collaboration between the Chief Medical Officer (CMO), Chief Nursing Officer (CNO), and Chief Operating Officer (COO), is gaining traction as a new method for optimising organisational performance in healthcare. Recognising the need for an integrated approach to leadership, this structure leverages the distinct C-suite expertise of medical, nursing, and operational executives.

The following case study is an example of this in action, *Hill J 2023,*

An acute hospital successfully leveraged triad leadership to reduce Central Line-Associated Blood Stream (CLABSI) Infections. The facility's COO, realising the significant impact of CLABSI rates on quality and financial outcomes, ensured the appropriate resourcing from an operational, financial, and human resource perspective. The CMO ensured that evidence-based medicine protocols were being followed and engaged in collaborative discussions with the medical staff. The CNO ensured daily infection control audits, conducted daily assessments with clinicians on the necessity for central lines, and completed a central line checklist at the time of insertion to monitor for sterility. In having this integrated and aligned approach to interventions, the hospital's focus was on expediting removal of unneeded central lines, limiting the use of temporary central lines, complying with best practice insertion techniques, strengthening central line maintenance, and promoting triad stewardship.

Results: A review of risk-adjusted data demonstrated the hospital had five CLABSI events in 2018, four in 2019, zero in 2020 and one CLABSI event in 2021.

Creating and maintaining a culture of safety requires management teams to demonstrate an ongoing commitment to prioritising patient safety measures. A patient-centred approach to fostering a just, transparent, and learning culture, that is embedded in the very fabric of the organisation requires ensuring non-punitive systems for reporting and learning from adverse events. Embedding safety culture team training into quality improvement projects, introducing programs that support a culture of escalation of concerns, and consistently supporting the front-line staff to identify, report, and rectify vulnerabilities in the clinical governance system, will strengthen the organisation's leadership capability to develop safe cultures.

1.6 Establishing a Clinical Governance System

Establishing or strengthening a clinical governance system can be a complex process; however, it is essential for ensuring that healthcare services are safe, effective, and of high quality. The following are key steps that leaders of health services can follow in establishing clinical governance systems within their organisations.

1. *Define the objective*: Determine what is needing to be achieved with your clinical governance system and set clear goals for improvement. This will help you to focus your efforts and ensure that you and your team are working towards a common purpose. This may be to either review one aspect of an existing system, to improve and strengthen the existing system in its entirety, or to create and embed each of the key components of clinical governance de novo.
2. *Assess the current system and conduct a gap analysis*: Conduct a comprehensive review of the current processes, policies, and procedures to identify any areas of weakness or potential risks. This step will inform the objectives you defined and allow for a good understanding of the overall perspective and scale of system redesign that is required.
3. *Develop policies and procedures*: Develop policies and procedures to support clinical governance, ensuring that they are consistent with best practices and relevant legislation and standards. These should include policies on patient safety, medical practitioner credentialing, risk management, and continuous improvement. It is crucial to conduct appropriate research and undertake external benchmarking to ensure alignment with relevant national and state legislative and regulatory requirements as well as contemporaneous practice. Benchmarking policies and procedures with those of peer health services and incorporating relevant expert clinician advice and review in their development is advised.
4. *Establish clinical governance committees*: Set up the foundational structure of clinical governance committees, consisting of relevant stakeholders, to oversee the implementation of your clinical governance system. The levels, sizes and reporting hierarchy of these committees will be informed by the unique context of your organisation and its challenges. These committees should be responsible for monitoring performance, assessing the quality of care, and making recommendations for improvement at a minimum. Relevant stakeholders should include representatives of appropriate seniority and experience from all key areas involved in the delivery of clinical care. Directors of Nursing, Senior Medical Practitioners, Clinical Risk Managers, Quality Managers, Perioperative Managers, and, where possible, a patient/consumer representative are suggested at a minimum, with the meetings chaired by a senior healthcare leader.
5. *Provide training and support*: Ensure that staff, including medical practitioners, receive the appropriate training and support they need to effectively implement the clinical governance system. This includes training on policies and procedures, facilitating external training sessions on the practice of clinical governance itself, providing relevant literature, guidelines, and standards, and opportunities for simulation training, and providing ongoing support and guidance to help staff continuously improve their skills and knowledge.
6. *Establish performance metrics*: Establish performance metrics to measure the effectiveness of your clinical governance system, including measures of patient safety, relevant clinical outcomes, quality of care, patient satisfaction, and staff engagement.

7. *Establish a clinical incident management system (CIMS)*: A CIMS is used to manage and report incidents and is a key component of a clinical governance system. The purpose of a CIMS is to identify, report, respond to, and prevent adverse events and to promote a culture of patient safety and continuous improvement. This enables the organisation to collect information about clinical incidents to determine causal and contributing factors, identify opportunities for improvement, and set up processes to immediately manage and respond to incidents, including assigning responsibilities and coordinating responses. In addition, this allows for the identification of trends and patterns over time, which can be reported and analysed to continuously improve the quality and safety of care provided.

   The capture and reporting of this data should align with external data reporting requirements and health service accreditation standards.
8. *Collect and analyse data*: Collect data on the performance of your clinical governance system using tools such as audits, surveys, and observational studies. Analyse this data to identify areas of strengths and weaknesses and to determine where improvements are needed. Mortality and morbidity reviews and clinical audits should be established as appropriate and designed to monitor the safe practice of the specific range of clinical services delivered within the staffing capacity and capability.
9. *Monitor and report on performance*: Report on the performance of your clinical governance system using the outcomes and incident data that is collected and analysed. This ensures there is transparency and accountability within the clinical governance system itself, and demonstrates the impact of clinical governance efforts. Reporting avenues will consist of those that are internal to the organisation and external, to governance agencies, databases, or clinical registries and for the purposes of benchmarking with peer organisations and against best-practice evidence. Providing this data to the public, community, and particularly future patients is an important part of clinical governance in terms of transparency. Public reporting is increasingly a feature of true consumer engagement and participation.
10. *Evaluate and continuously improve*: Continuously review and improve your clinical governance system, ensuring that it remains effective and relevant as your organisation evolves.

By following these steps, healthcare leaders can set up an elementary yet robust clinical governance system that will help to ensure that the healthcare services provided by the organisation for which they are accountable are safe, effective, and of high quality.

1.7 Role of Hospital Accreditation

In Australia and across the world, various forms of independent and standardised accreditation of health organisations exist, the purpose of which is to provide some level of assurance to the community that the health service meets expected patient safety and quality of care standards.

Hospital accreditation involves an assessment by qualified external peer reviewers to evaluate a health service's compliance against predetermined quality and safety standards, with the aim of improving healthcare quality and promoting ongoing quality improvement. Generally, all public and private hospitals, as well as day procedure services and most public dental practices, are required to be accredited in order to continue to operate. As an example, the *Australian Commission on Safety and Quality in Health Care (ACSQHC)* coordinates this national process via assessment against the set requirements of the *National Safety and Quality Health Service (NSQHS) Standards* in Australia.

Accreditation is viewed as a reputable tool to evaluate and enhance the quality of healthcare, and there is a reasonable amount of evidence to support this notion, particularly that compliance with accreditation standards has positive associations with improving the safety culture, efficiency, patient lengths of stay, and process-related performance measures.

The mandatory and cyclical nature of accreditation has raised the issue of it being viewed primarily as a regulatory and compliance goal, as opposed to the intended objective of engagement and commitment to continuous quality improvement. This can result in the focus of accreditation being a task-based project to ensure the correct paperwork and frameworks are drafted and presented ahead of an accreditation visit. An entire industry of quality coordinators and accreditation project officers has developed as a result, which assists greatly in meeting the workload of accreditation. However, this practice has been observed to risk disconnection with and disempowerment of front-line staff in owning or being accountable for creating practical and sustained quality solutions relevant to their areas.

In an endeavour to move away from this idea of an 'orchestrated, choreographed accreditation event' where it can be argued that such a temporary façade has the potential to inadvertently bury the real issues, Australia and other jurisdictions have instituted a 'short-notice accreditation' process. This is based on the premise that accreditation certification needs to be embedded in the 'business as usual' model of health services, and ownership for improving quality needs to be an ongoing focus, for which everyone is responsible.

A short-notice mandatory assessment may occur at any time and at least once during an accreditation cycle. Health services are given 24 hours of notice, i.e., one business day or other similar 'short notice' of an upcoming assessment.

In general, the assessment process includes interviews with staff, observation of operational and clinical areas, review of documents, and examination of how systems are used to reduce risks and improve safety. Following an assessment, there is a remediation period afforded to the health service to implement any improvements identified and/or to demonstrate compliance with any actions that may not have met the required criteria during the initial assessment.

Health leaders are advised to ensure that there are active and continuous processes in place at their organisations to support ongoing quality improvement and to meet new assessment requirements.

A process of *continuous* self-assessment against the requirements of accreditation standards will be beneficial at all levels of an organisation.

Involvement of patients or consumers, the community, and relevant external stakeholders is also important in preparing for external evaluation processes as well as in the designing of internal quality and safety governance systems.

Further Reading

Hill J Jr, Carlucci AM. Overview of Triad Leadership. Healthcare Administration Leadership & Management Journal. (2025);3(1)16/20.

Hill J Jr, Manzo J, Ramic M, et al. Central line associated blood stream infection reduction at an academic community hospital during the COVID-19 pandemic to achieve patient safety. Physician Leadership Journal. 2023;10(3):16-23.

Byrnes J and Teman S. The Safety Playbook: a healthcare leader's guide to building a high-reliability organisation. 2018.

Braithwaite J and Travaglia Joanne F (2008) An overview of clinical governance policies, practices and initiatives. Australian Health Review 32, 10–22.

VMIA, strengthening clinical governance for health service boards, 2015.

ACHS, National Safety and Quality Health Service (NSQHS) Standards, 2021. Second edition.

Delivering High Quality Healthcare – Victorian Clinical Governance Framework: Department of Health Victoria (2017).

National Safety and Quality Health Service Standards, Australian Commission on Safety and Quality in Health Care (2011).

Hussein, M., Pavlova, M., Ghalwash, M. *et al.* The impact of hospital accreditation on the quality of healthcare: a systematic literature review. *BMC Health Serv Res* **21**, 1057 (2021). https://doi.org/10.1186/s12913-021-07097-6

Health care accreditation and quality of care: exploring the role of accreditation and external evaluation of health care facilities and organisations. Geneva: World Health Organisation; 2022. Licence: CC BY-NC-SA 3.0 IGO.

Barnett, ML, Olenski, AR & Jena, AB 2017, 'Patient Mortality During Unannounced Accreditation Surveys at US Hospitals', JAMA Intern Med, vol. 177, no. 5, pp. 693–700

Australian Health and Hospitals Association. Short-Notice Accreditation Assessment Pilot. Accessed via https://ahha.asn.au/sites/default/files/docs/policy-issue/short_notice_accreditation_assessment_pilot.pdf

Australian Commission on Safety and Quality in Health Care 2023. Fact sheet 17: Short notice accreditation assessment. Accessed via https://www.safetyandquality.gov.au/sites/default/files/2023-10/fact_sheet_17_short_notice_accreditation_assessment.pdf

https://www.safetyandquality.gov.au/standards/nsqhs-standards/assessment-nsqhs-standards/consumers-and-accreditation#:~:text=Accreditation%20is%20an%20evaluation%20process,safe%20and%20high%20quality%20healthcare

Hill J Jr, Carlucci AM. Overview of Triad Leadership. Healthcare Administration Leadership & Management Journal. (2025);3(1)16/20.

2 Leadership in Clinical Governance

Effective leadership is critical for successful clinical governance. It requires a multifaceted approach, encompassing not only strategic vision, but also the ability to foster a culture of continuous improvement and accountability. Leaders must champion transparency in reporting, ensuring data-driven decision-making, and promoting open dialogue around performance. This involves empowering clinicians to actively participate in governance processes, and facilitating a shared understanding of quality standards and patient safety protocols. Furthermore, leadership in this context necessitates the proactive identification of risks and the implementation of effective mitigation strategies, constantly adapting to evolving best practices and regulatory requirements.

Ultimately, strong leadership is the linchpin that transforms clinical governance from a compliance exercise into a dynamic process for enhancing patient outcomes. Various organisational structures for clinical governance exist in healthcare. What follows is a description that can be applied to either an individual healthcare facility, such as a hospital, or indeed across an entire healthcare system.

There is no one correct method of how an organisational structure that is conducive to good clinical governance should be constructed. What is required, however, is clarity as to the specific responsibilities and accountabilities for clinical governance within the organisation, and therefore, the establishment of clear reporting lines at each level. This allows issues and concerns to be escalated appropriately in a timely manner where staff can be provided with easy access to those responsible for the direction of quality and safety.

The board and executive accountabilities for clinical governance have been described in the previous chapter. With regard to reporting responsibilities to and from the executive, the committee structure should have scope for the formation of a peak body that holds overarching accountability for clinical governance across the facility or system. The peak or highest level of clinical governance oversight is usually led by the clinical executive (CMO and/or CNO) responsible for clinical governance within the organisation. This multidisciplinary group/committees reporting to

© The Author(s), under exclusive license to Springer Nature Singapore Pte Ltd. 2026
L. Prado, S. Chandrasiri, *The Practice of Clinical Governance*,
https://doi.org/10.1007/978-981-19-7896-8_2

the executive should have clear terms of reference, agenda, and reporting in terms of clinical governance.

The peak clinical governance committee commonly comprises a multidisciplinary membership with clearly articulated terms of reference and work plans. Key areas of focus for this group should include the development and revision of the organisation's safety and quality strategy, clinical governance framework, relevant high-level policies and procedures, and the monitoring of key clinical governance indicators. Determining targeted improvement programs or specific actions in response to outcome variations, and ensuring compliance with the implementation of these throughout the organisation should be a main purpose. The peak committee should also ensure there are processes in place for the escalation of emerging clinical concerns and risks to patient care, such as safety alerts. In addition, significant clinical incidents, the management of those incidents, and the progress towards resolution should be monitored by this group. Consumer representation and patient engagement at this level are critical.

To aid in setting the tone and fostering a patient-centred safety culture, when managers and executive meet to discuss operational issues, they should consider the use of patient incidents and reflections of events that have occurred to patients over the previous 24 hours, or since their last meeting, as the initial essential indicators of performance at the meeting. For example, a daily huddle, whether it's conducted at the unit, team, or facility level, should start with a reflection or description of any incidents to patients and patient care issues of concern. This highlights the importance of patient safety to all members and sets the foundation, or higher purpose of the meeting.

By commencing with an overview of patient incidents, this ensures any outstanding issues that are yet to be resolved for individual patients who have been harmed or have suffered from injury in the previous 24 hours or since the last meeting, are rectified as soon as possible. In addition, the opportunity for any other rectification or notification of safety alerts to other members of the organisation to prevent similar incidents of harm, can occur at this time.

Executive and managers, including those with non-clinical backgrounds, must lead by example and proactively ask for reports on patient incidents and outcomes at or ahead of these meetings. Similarly, formal reporting of patient incidents through an incident management/reporting system will automatically trigger alerts to the appropriate managers requesting relevant responses, within the shortest time possible. Ensuring that incident-related queries are resolved early, investigations commenced, and patient harm mitigated under a patient-centric model, is practically driven by the management team by making appropriate enquiries following the receipt of incident reports.

To demonstrate an organisational commitment to clinical governance, the executive can formally acknowledge the contribution of staff in patient safety. This formal recognition may take the form of reward and recognition programs or other acknowledgement of staff performance and innovation in care and patient safety. Formal recognition of clinical governance and staff contributions in patient safety activities within an organisation is essential in setting the tone of the organisation's values, tolerance, and attitude towards the importance of a patient-centred safety culture.

Investing in supporting and enabling staff to engage in focused and ongoing professional development in clinical governance is an important aspect of recognising the importance of this in professional practice.

Encouraging and facilitating the introduction of projects focused on the development of new systems and policies for safe service delivery, and considering local investment or budget allocations for supporting business cases targeted at making improvements or efficiencies in how care is delivered, are foundational actions that the executive can undertake in setting the appropriate tone within the organisation. Similarly, research in clinical governance, although complex, should be considered, particularly in larger organisations, as part of the organisation's overarching research strategy. Doing so elevates the academic prowess for evidence-based clinical governance practice, and consequently its importance within the organisation as well as the broader healthcare sector.

2.1 Role of the Board

Effective clinical governance requires clear and direct '*lines of sight*' from the frontline patient-clinician interactions, whether at the bedside, in the operating theatre, or at a clinic, right through to the level of the health service board (governing body). This ensures that fundamental elements of clinical governance are in place from a day-to-day operational level through to high-level oversight and allows for the continuous monitoring and evaluation of performance. With these building blocks firmly embedded, early identification of unwarranted variations, predictive analysis of emerging trends and undertaking comparative analysis with peer benchmarking, enable rapid responses and timely interventions to be actioned and improvements to be planned.

A shared understanding of the importance of clinical governance in the healthcare system is key to ensuring that patients are safe, clinicians are safe, and that hospitals are safe.

The following section will explore the standard organisational roles and structures that are conducive to facilitating this 'line of sight', to equip and empower all healthcare leaders who are responsible for clinical governance undertake their respective responsibilities in a clear and transparent manner.

The governing body, usually the 'board', sets the overall strategy of the organisation and therefore, by direct extension, the tone, expectation and standard of safety and quality for patient care. All board members are required to have a comprehensive understanding of their clinical governance responsibilities that is at a minimum, equivalent to the understanding of their financial, legal, and corporate accountabilities for the organisation.

The board should also expect to be well-versed and familiar with the status and challenges of the culture of the organisation with respect to safety and quality. As clinical care can often be complex for non-clinicians to understand, it is advisable that board members learn and upskill together, to have a shared understanding of how clinical services are provided and therefore how outcomes can be assessed, monitored, and improved.

It is important that board members balance the scrutiny of, and accountability for, clinical outcomes with financial outcomes of their organisation, employing a 'values-based' or similar outcome-driven sustainability perspective, and allow for considered, meaningful, and appropriate fiscal viability within the organisation. Whilst the prevailing tendency for boards has been to prioritise financial viability of an organisation first and foremost, it is important to note that many recent examples of significant clinical governance failures in Australia and around the world have, following investigation, in fact, identified fundamental failures of board governance and oversight for patient safety, as having been the primary contributing factor.

This therefore necessitates an in-depth exploration of 'how' boards can and should undertake this responsibility. To begin with, a focus on education, training, and professional competency development in clinical governance for boards is essential and should encompass the following key areas that the board should understand:

1. *What* clinical services are delivered across the organisation and *why*.
2. *How* these clinical services determine the metrics that need to be measured, and to what degree safety and quality performance is tracked in the organisation's clinical services plan.

The board needs to ensure that the clinical services plan integrates financial metrics, workforce indicators, operational outcomes, and performance indicators, with clinical outcomes and safety and quality measures that have been identified as appropriate reflectors of success in the delivery of their services. With increasing frequency, we are seeing many occasions of new clinical services and cutting-edge technologies being introduced under the guise of 'innovation', without due diligence or consideration having been given for establishing relevant performance and outcome measures to evaluate their impact.

The board needs to ensure that all new clinical services have firstly, been considered from a balanced perspective, and needs to be aware that success cannot be measured only by financial profitability. When considering the development, expansion, or review of clinical services, the board should initially question the capacity and capability of the facility to undertake the relevant service. This is particularly important when established services may not be performing to expected clinical outcome standards or delivering expected profit margins.

Capacity relates to whether and to what degree there is a clinical need for the service within the community served, and whether and to what degree that need can realistically be met, in terms of infrastructure (beds), workforce (staff and doctors), capital assets (equipment), and other resources. As an example, consider the situation of an organisation wishing to commence a new maternity service. Commencing and providing safe service requires specialist staffing, including sub-specialised areas such neonatal anaesthesia or IVF (in-vitro fertilisation) specialists. A mismatch in the scope and capacity of the service being planned, with that of the obstetric needs of the community can lead to a service commencing with significant pressure from the outset, both in terms of financial performance and in the safety and quality of care that can be provided. Even if initial capacity can be managed with sufficient resources, people, equipment, and beds, each of these requires commitment to guarantee ongoing supply and availability to the same or a higher level. Therefore, the board needs to approach what may initially seem like a quick win, by asking some pertinent questions as to whether there is current capacity and, if not, then how and from where this capacity is being created so as to be assured that a service that is commenced is done so safely. The board should ask about the 'must have' essential components of 'capacity' that need to be in place.

Capability refers to the ability to safely provide the primary service in terms of what other secondary or support services are required. This includes the specific requirements for clinicians to be experienced in particular areas of clinical practice. For example, to introduce a bone marrow transplant service, whilst there may be 'capacity', it is important that key secondary services, such as intensive care, emergency medicine, infectious diseases, and support services such as pathology, radiology, and pharmacy are available to support the primary service. The staff involved need to be credentialed to be able to provide this service safely, effectively, and efficiently. Specific training, education, policies, and procedures to guide operations, including clinical pathways and clinical guidelines need to be in place. Therefore, the board needs to enquire about the broader capability of the organisation to sufficiently meet these requirements, beyond just the capacity to provide the planned service.

The board should further question how capability has been determined, the nature of the gap analysis that has been undertaken, and the strategies that have been considered or are being put in place to address any deficiencies.

Reviewing capacity and capability is a vital part of the risk analysis function of service planning and informs the board as to whether the particular service being planned or delivered is safe. It is helpful for board members to hear from senior clinicians who will be directly involved in service delivery, particularly in the introduction of a new service. The enthusiasm that can often be brought to the board by clinicians must of course be tempered, as it can make open discussion of the reality of key safety concerns difficult. To provide this balance, board membership should include individuals with a high-level understanding of clinical governance and the delivery of healthcare.

In addition, the board should have clear and regular access to the executive with accountability for clinical governance and service delivery, such as the chief medical officer/chief nursing officer equivalents.

2.1.1 Board Review of Safety and Quality Indicators

The board needs to confirm the indicators that will be utilised in monitoring and evaluating the services, to provide a level of assurance in the safety and quality outputs of the organisation. In determining the list of such indicators, board members need to ensure that they have a good understanding of which indicators provide overall assurance of quality, and which indicators provide a more 'sensitive' or 'specific' assurance of quality trends and variances. Detecting such trends and unexpected deviations ought to alert the board to request further information in order to obtain a better understanding of the drivers and tools that would then be required to counter these changes.

A dashboard that provides clear identification of any variation or changes in the indicators is very useful. Choosing which indicators are relevant and meaningful is a complex undertaking, and therefore the board should be inquiring *'why'* certain indicators are chosen by the executive and *'how'* these indicators are actually impacted. The key question the board needs to understand and ask is, ***'how does this tell us if the service is safe?'***

Other indicators, such as patient experience measures, cultural staff surveys, numbers of complaints and compliments, etc., also play an important role in the overall assessment by the board.

When selecting and having oversight over clinical indicators, the board should be prioritising those which reflect high-risk clinical services, such as, for example, maternity and mental health services. In addition to monitoring the indicators of these clinical services, the board should consider commissioning a regular review of the key high-risk clinical services as part of the safety and quality plan and internal audit program. For example, a 'rolling plan' for the review of services (e.g. maternity services clinical review every 2–3 years) ensures that even if a service appears to be performing well, a thorough investigation of its clinical practice, outcomes, benchmarking data, consideration of new, changed, or expired equipment, service delivery models, etc., can provide a platform for continuous improvement, and can set the tone for a culture of organisational improvement.

The board is advised to ask input from consumers of healthcare within their organisation and to consider director positions on the board being made available to consumers. A strong representation of consumers on board subcommittees, and on other peak committees within the organisation, particularly those involved in safety and quality, is strongly recommended, as is having patient experience measures monitored as a routine Board KPI (key performance indicator).

The board should consider establishing a formal subcommittee dedicated to the high-level oversight of patient care, clinical governance, and safety and quality, which can provide for thorough investigation and monitoring of the clinical governance performance of the organisation. It should have as its members people with extensive *practical* experience in clinical governance. The organisation's executive who are accountable for clinical governance should be expected to routinely present to this committee and provide detail with regard to the performance of the clinical governance system.

In setting a tone of safety and quality, the board should consider by which mechanism it will be formally advised on serious adverse events, and how it can be assured that subsequent investigations, recommendations, and actions will be implemented and followed through. The board can also set the tone by having the patient voice 'heard' at board level, for example via the inclusion of patient stories specifically with an emphasis on when harm has occurred. Finally, by choosing to meet staff and patients directly, and by regularly 'rounding' through the organisation to hear the voice from the ground level and at the front line of clinical practice, the board sends a clear message that they consider patient safety as being paramount.

In developing and approving the overall strategy of the organisation, the board needs to ensure that safety and quality, and patient experience make up a significant component of the strategy, and are aligned with the values and purpose of the organisation. There should be clarity on how clinical governance will actually be achieved through the strategy, how clinical governance will impact and be impacted by the services provided, how the clinical governance strategy 'frames' the clinical services strategy, and how it will facilitate the setting of the overarching 'tone' for patient safety across the organisation.

Clear improvement plans outlining how clinical governance will be delivered, should further make up part of the strategy or be closely aligned to the strategy through specific operational plans, with clear performance indicators and the accountabilities for monitoring these made clear, as described above.

Much discussion and debate currently exist regarding which indicators of clinical governance a board should use to monitor and therefore provide oversight for. What is crucial, is that all board members understand how an indicator is produced or arises, how it is impacted, and how it reflects safety and quality. Regardless of which indicators are selected, it is each board members' responsibility to be sufficiently educated and trained to ensure a deep understanding of the indicators, including external benchmarking, trending of results, and drivers of change.

A practical way the board can set the tone for ensuring that clinical governance is delivered in a patient-centric manner, is by delegating permissions to management to respond appropriately and quickly when a significant clinical incident occurs. This includes permission for the provision of an apology, without fearing legal consequences, and offering out-of-pocket expense reimbursements to patients and their families who may have been harmed. Such endorsement by the board of when to undertake proactive measures in incident management sets a clear tone of patient-centric care and a focus on safety and quality.

2.2 The Role of Leaders

Leaders need to pose this question to themselves: *'As a leader, what is the most frustrating thing that I have done that impacts on clinicians?'*

And clinicians need to ask themselves: *'What is the most frustrating thing I do that impacts on administrators/leaders?'*

Characteristics of good leadership in clinical governance include clarity of purpose, sustaining the vision for others, building trust and credibility in the organisation, being persistent when challenged by obstacles, working with and through others with a 'service' approach in mind, freely giving praise, having keen self-awareness, and being formally educated in healthcare executive management.

Leaders need to commit to their own continuous professional development in healthcare across all domains. They need to reflect on their own professional and emotional responses to crises, emergencies, and significant clinical incidents. They need to use research and education in clinical governance as levers for clinician engagement, know how their hospital and healthcare system works, be present on the ground with teams and be 'visible' throughout the organisation.

Leaders need to be relentless in the pursuit of quality improvement, and 'obsessed with failure' so that failure is not replicated. They need to be transparent with results and performance, proactively engage clinicians, staff, and those on the front line, and be *'person-centred'* with an authentic emphasis on patients. And finally, they must have the determination and drive to lead and be part of a *high-reliability organisation*.

There are often several particular barriers to strong clinician engagement, as clinicians may feel overwhelmed, ill-equipped, and/or may have limited understanding of how their behaviour contributes to safety and quality in healthcare. Leaders, and those who pay for healthcare, tend to often focus only on financial and non-clinical indicators, and therefore must be conscious that this is often a major barrier to clinicians being engaged.

Organisations often have obstacles in *sustaining* a culture of continuous quality improvement, where administrative decisions can seem to be disassociated from the practicalities of patient care. Policies and processes can seem more important than outcomes, and the principal focus on financial metrics over patient care indicators can create significant barriers and disconnect with the clinicians. A particularly critical obstacle when trying to engage staff and doctors is the lack of transparency and accountability for performance in clinical governance. It is therefore vital that leaders use valid and reliable data to frame and demonstrate how patient safety and overall clinical governance is delivered and maintained throughout the organisation.

Leaders can work diligently to create a culture of patient safety by personally committing to upholding high standards of quality, ensuring that clinicians are embedded within the leadership structure of the organisation, and providing training to those clinicians who are in leadership roles. Their role is to ensure the workplace is psychologically safe for staff, particularly in terms of a 'just' culture, and to encourage 'speaking up' when they see patient safety breaches.

Leaders create the culture of patient safety by leading by example, driving the vision, and engaging colleagues and other clinicians in patient safety. Being open and honest in communications and dialogue, particularly when rounding with staff, doctors, and patients, is critical to creating a safe and high-functioning culture. Responding to the ideas and needs of clinicians ensures their voice is heard, that they feel they are being engaged, and that they are provided the opportunity to impact on decisions that are made throughout the organisation.

Delivery of patient care is complicated and resource intensive. Therefore, unnecessary barriers should be removed where possible, so that the delivery of care is as straightforward and streamlined for staff members and clinical teams as much as possible. It is important for clinicians to know that they can have confidence in the management team of the hospital, and that the hospital administrators are capable of carrying out their duties. A key way of ensuring and demonstrating this, is by ensuring ongoing two-way, transparent communication between clinicians and hospital administrators, which is fundamental to the success of the organisation.

The executive, particularly the clinical executive, has responsibility for setting the tone for ongoing innovation, education, and training in clinical governance. In addition to regular forums for staff that provide opportunities for ongoing learning, the clinical executive can ensure other aspects of clinical governance are also included on a regular basis as part of the training and education programs for all staff. Using patient stories, case examples, and case studies, will enable staff to be involved in the education and learning about patient safety from a practical perspective. They can be included in panels, debates, in sharing learnings across different campuses, and other team-based learning opportunities. Setting a tone of education and training across the organisation can influence the process of learning that occurs at the clinical unit level among colleagues as well.

Case-based learning across the organisation at the unit level can provide opportunities for ongoing reflective practice, in terms of understanding and analysing what went well and what did not go well when an incident occurs. This is an important way of ensuring that opportunities for ongoing improvement occurs at the individual clinician and team level.

2.3 The Role of Staff

Whilst clinicians have a major role in the clinical governance initiatives at a hospital, all staff, regardless of their varying duties, have a role in supporting clinical governance, safety, and quality within their organisations. Therefore, it is important that all staff are familiar with the basic elements of clinical governance.

As an example, 'porters/orderlies', who are responsible for patient transport, need to be aware that in the event of patient deterioration during transport, they know how to access assistance immediately. Staff involved in cleaning, catering, and other patient assistance roles also need to have an understanding of the elements of safety and quality as they apply to the roles they perform within the organisation.

All managers should understand how their teams impact on patient care, and particularly how they themselves can play a role in improving the quality of patient outcomes. Therefore, education and training in clinical governance needs to align with all roles within an organisation.

Patient safety is everyone's business and ensuring that education and training are pitched at the right levels, so that staff feel they have clarity on how they can assist in situations of ensuring patient safety, even if their roles are non-clinical, is critical.

2.4 Role of the C-Suite

The executive or C-suite of a healthcare organisation play several critical roles in ensuring that clinical governance is practiced at the highest level across an organisation. Like the board, healthcare executives need to ensure that they are well trained and educated, with a good understanding of the elements of clinical governance. Importantly, all executive should have an understanding of how clinical governance is practiced in their organisation, how it is monitored, and how outcomes can be improved.

Leading this at the executive or C-suite level are usually the roles of the CMO/CNO or equivalents. Whilst all executives have a role in clinical governance, the 'clinical' executives have the most significant roles and will usually hold *executive responsibility* for clinical governance within the organisation.

In addition to being the subject matter experts on the topic, the clinical executives need to work closely with other non-clinical executives to ensure that there is a 'shared' understanding of the importance of clinical governance. They need to assist the non-clinical executives in understanding and preparing for their roles in clinical governance in terms of how they can then work together with the clinical executives to influence the manner in which clinical governance is practiced throughout the organisation.

The clinical executive must ensure that they are well across the developments, innovations, evidence, new research, and changes in clinical governance practices at an international and national level. They should ensure that appropriate national and international benchmarks are used to address the organisation's performance. By sharing patient stories and the impact on patients when harm occurs, with the whole executive team, the clinical executives set the tone at the highest level on how the organisation can provide safe clinical services whilst balancing financial and other performance measures.

In the same way that non-clinical executives need to understand operational performance such as activity, revenue, margin, labour, and other costs, they must also understand clinical governance, so that they can speak to and be aware of the impact of clinical governance on the operational performance of the organisation. Similarly, the clinical executives need to understand the 'cost' of harm from both an operational perspective to the organisation, as well as from an individual patient level. Taking a 'value-based' perspective in the delivery of clinical services can provide an effective approach to ensuring a good balance between clinical and financial outcomes.

In addition to the delivery of clinical governance within the organisation, the clinical executive also sets the tone in terms of research, innovation, training, and education in clinical governance. An organisation that is leading in clinical governance will have active programs in education and training where safety and quality make up key components. Examples of this include how incidents are to be reviewed within a 'just culture' framework and what investigation 'tools' are to be used, and programs for developing communication skills with respect to speaking up for patient safety, including ensuring staff understand that they feel supported to do so.

Education and training in understanding clinical governance indicators, how they relate to performance, how they are measured, and how they can be improved, are crucial. Education and training in key policies, procedures, and processes that provide a safe environment for patients, such as how to recognise and escalate clinical deterioration, perform appropriate clinical assessments of patients as required, and the application of programs targeted at the prevention of patient harm, are also required.

The clinical executive must ensure that these education and training programs are ongoing however, and are not just provided as a 'one-off' occurrence done at the time of 'onboarding' for example, as this is often undertaken only when a new staff member joins the organisation.

The executive can set the tone for patient safety right from the start at the onboarding process, where they can use patient stories to establish the standards and expectations for the delivery of clinical care, and how outcomes of care are to be monitored. New staff should be made aware of how the 'just culture' in the organisation is actually practiced from a practical perspective. As an example, if the organisation is committed to open disclosure, then open disclosure should be explained at onboarding sessions so that all new staff understand their respective roles in open disclosure, as well as being provided appropriate mentoring/assistance in how they are expected to deliver such a key clinical governance program. New staff need to understand how clinical governance forms part of the overarching organisational strategy and how it aligns with the organisation's purpose and values.

Executives should ensure these staff have access to ongoing training after commencement, through regular forums and similar information sessions. These can include traditional formal sessions where specific clinical governance information is shared, e.g. introducing new clinical governance policies and procedures that are being implemented across the organisation. However, informal sessions such as 'open forums', 'clinical councils' and similar structures however named, must also be enabled, as these allow for free dialogue and discussion between staff, management and executives, which leads to a better shared understanding of the challenges and opportunities, and allows concerns to be raised effectively.

What is critical at either type of forum is including the voice of the patient and the consumer by enabling their engagement and active participation at each level of the organisation where possible. The patient's voice can be 'heard' through the telling of patient stories to set the tone of the discussion, or indeed if possible, having patients and their families, along with other consumers, present their stories themselves at these forum. Patients and their families, participating directly in such discussions and even in leading these discussions, can be of great benefit.

Often, the findings resulting from investigations into failures of clinical governance can focus significantly on apparent poor leadership, which particularly reflects the lack of clarity with respect to board and executive accountability and responsibility for clinical governance. As described, board and chief executive officer responsibility for clinical governance is key, however, all members of the executive and C-suite have important roles to play in this regard.

C-suite executives usually have responsibility specific to a particular area of expertise, such as human resources, information technology, or finance, with accountability for clinical governance resting specifically with the clinical executives. However, as 'the provision of clinical care' is the core business of all hospitals and healthcare organisations, it is critical that all members of the C-suite and their respective teams understand their key roles in supporting, directly and indirectly, clinical governance in their organisation.

When organisations are struggling from a financial performance perspective, it is often a common response for the C-suite to come together to clearly identify the issues and determine an action plan moving forward. All C-suite executives are expected to understand core financial indicators and drivers and participate in the remedial actions necessary. Fundamentally, C-suite members should be considered *healthcare executives* first, and subject matter experts second. This reflects the expectation that all C-suite members are expected to understand financial performance measures, the levers that direct change, and ensure their teams are involved in the improvement plans. In responding to a financial challenge then, the C-suite would jointly work on a plan for improving the operational performance. Focal areas in these scenarios often include and will look at the management of costs, the management of labour, improving activity, and expanding clinical activity.

Common financial key performance indicators (KPIs) for C-suite executives are as follows:

- Management of labour costs:
  - Labour hours per patient day
  - Hourly labour rate
  - Labour costs per operating suite
- Management of activity:
  - Length of stay (LOS)
  - Revenue per patient day
  - Theatre utilisation %
  - Emergency department presentation to admission conversion rate
- Management of other costs:
  - Pharmacy cost per admission
  - Medical consumables per admission
  - Costs per operating minute
- Expanding clinical activity:
  - % growth of clinical areas, e.g. overnight admissions and same day admissions.
- Financial management:
  - EBITDA
  - Capex expenditure

Whilst the detail of these KPIs remains the remit of the specific subject matter expert C-suite executive, such as the CFO, all C-suite executives still require at least a basic understanding of these drivers and how they can be influenced, as they will have a role in managing or assisting with managing these drivers. In addition, and not uncommonly, all executives are required to make difficult decisions to sometimes rapidly improve the overall financial situation. This may include reducing staffing costs and discretionary costs such as training, education, functions, and conferences. Individual executives are responsible for their portfolio budgets and staffing, and are often incentivised for contributing to improving the operational and financial performance of the organisation, in terms of their own remuneration.

In all businesses, executives are also generally expected to have a good understanding of the key indicators of the 'product/service' that is provided by their particular organisation. This specifically includes indicators that reflect the quality standard or quality performance of the product/service being delivered, as this indicates the overall performance and success of the organisation, for which all executives are ultimately responsible. They are expected to therefore know how the quality indicators are influenced, monitored, reported and how they influence the financial performance of the business.

In healthcare, this main 'service/product' is the clinical care or service that is provided to a patient. The financial performance of a healthcare organisation therefore depends very much on the standard of quality of the service that is provided. However, as not all executives of healthcare organisations are often across the safety and quality indicators of their clinical services and how these indicators are performing, they are therefore not able to impact and improve the financial and overall performance of the organisation.

Ownership of the clinical quality indicators and responsibility for how these indicators are performing usually sit primarily with the 'clinical' executives, e.g. Chief Medical Officer (CMO) and Chief Nursing Officer (CNO). Whilst this is understandable, it is essential, for the reasons outlined above, that all executives understand the safety and quality indicators, how they are influenced, the risks to the organisation if the indicators do not perform as expected, and how the indicators relate to the financial situation of the organisation.

The consequent impact of poorly performing quality indicators on the financial position may be significant and may even lead to staff layoffs, cost-cutting, and realignment of business models. These are significant impacts, where the business (healthcare service) itself could even face risk of closure or reduction in services.

Whilst poorly performing quality indicators could lead to significant operational business risks as outlined above, there are also additional serious consequences in the *business* of healthcare. Poorly performing quality indicators can reflect poor clinical outcomes that directly impact the actual health and wellbeing of individual human beings—the patients. Poor clinical outcomes can also lead to significant impacts on teams and individual staff members, particularly clinicians, who themselves hold individual professional accountability and responsibility for clinical care, including to regulatory agencies which may also overlap with medico-legal consequences.

Therefore, all executives in healthcare should ensure that they understand:

- The clinical quality indicators that reflect the performance of their healthcare organisation,
- Their role in the clinical governance program that oversees these indicators,
- The risks to the organisation if these indicators are performing poorly, and
- The implications and degree of potential harm that these risks present to patients, families, communities, and staff/clinicians.

To ensure this level of understanding and oversight exists within and across the executives and whole C-suite team, there needs to be a commitment by the board and executive leadership to ensuring they uphold a fundamental understanding of their respective roles in clinical governance. For this to be successful and as described, the board and CEO must lead by firstly setting the tone and by influencing the culture of the organisation in clinical governance. Most healthcare organisations have vision and mission statements, purpose outlines, and a list of values that speaks of a commitment to quality in clinical care in some manner, e.g. '*excellence*', '*world's best*', or '*leading*'. It must be realised that these committments cannot be truly upheld by just words written down in strategy documents if the organisation wishes to be successful in the core business it delivers.

If clinical governance indicators, and therefore clinical performance, are seen to be essential to the board and the CEO, they can then influence the remainder of the C-suite. There are several ways that the board and the CEO can set the tone and lead the executives in this regard.

2.5 Executive Involvement in Clinical Governance

The rationale for ensuring an understanding of clinical governance and outcomes can be fundamentally and easily demonstrated by using the analogy of the rationale for understanding financial indicators of any business. However, often this is set aside, with the argument being made that clinical outcomes are 'too complicated' and therefore need to remain within the remits of the CMO/CNO's expertise alone.

As described above, the C-suite or executive cannot simply exempt themselves from the consequences of 'poorly performing' quality indicators by citing that it is 'clinical stuff'. They must accept that their roles and their teams will need to still have involvement in the 'clinical stuff', because in most circumstances the 'clinical stuff' may be critical to the financial and operational success of the healthcare organisation itself.

It is important to note the true impact of the board and executive leadership on the culture of an organisation. If the board and executive not only know the clinical governance performance of the organisation, but also understands the drivers behind the indicators, such as the 'human' impact and how the success of the organisation is so closely related to these indicators, then their influence can be widespread and significant. It is important to note that this not only impacts the reputation of the organisation but can also have a great impact on staff, particularly clinical staff, whose professional motivations and 'sense of self' are very often closely tied to both their individual clinical performance as well as the organisation's overall clinical performance. This relates to the clinician's individual professional drivers such as their sense of a duty of care for improving the lives of others, and 'doing the best they can' for their patients. Therefore, learning and demonstrating these indicators, and more importantly the standard of care that these indicators reflect, is an important challenge for the board and the CEO. In addition to 'knowing' and 'understanding' the outcomes and performance of the organisation, highlighting the standards of quality performance in board reports, sharing patient and clinical stories, focusing on questioning the data that is presented, and asking for detailed explanations in relation to clinical governance performance information that they are presented with, are all examples of how a board can demonstrate a culture of safety. Alternative approaches can also include for example, commencing relevant meetings by firstly acknowledging clinical governance performance in relevant areas before proceeding to relate other non-clinical indicators with that of clinical governance performance, e.g., demonstrating how an increase in hospital-acquired infections may result in an increase in expenditure and therefore impact revenue and the financial bottom line of the entire department or organisation.

If all executives are well-versed in clinical governance, they are then able to influence the behaviour and actions of their own non-clinical teams. Therefore, when these teams are interacting with clinicians and clinical support staff, they will have a better understanding of the motivations and decisions of clinicians and the stressors they face, as well as the impacts of poor clinical governance performance.

Clinicians can be significantly impacted by clinical governance failures whether they relate to an individual patient (e.g. an unexpected death) or to a system-wide issue such as medication errors. The impact on staff performance in these situations from a clinical governance perspective is greatly influenced by the behaviour and interactions between staff, in addition to the financial pressures from the organisation (that could result in a reduction of rostered staff) and/or a lack of investment in capital (resulting in not being able to upgrade or replace essential clinical equipment).

By understanding, or at least acknowledging these complex social, psychological, and professional factors that challenge clinical staff, executives will be able to perform better in their roles and appropriately exert their influence across the organisation. In addition, as executives in healthcare hold a broader degree of accountability and responsibility for patient and staff safety which extends beyond just their own specific portfolios, this can often challenge them in a manner unlike their counterparts in non-healthcare organisations.

2.5.1 Chief People Officer (CPO)

The head of human resources, people and culture, is traditionally seen as a very distinct subject matter expertise role, focusing on industrial relations, union relationships, position descriptions, and performance management. It's relatively straightforward to understand the CPO role as it relates to workforce planning, professional development, enterprise bargaining, and workplace psychosocial and occupational safety. Whilst healthcare has unique challenges in these areas, experienced healthcare workforce HR teams are accustomed to dealing with these. Workplace diversity, cultural diversity, and equal opportunity employment are also familiar areas for the HR teams.

The greatest challenge for HR in healthcare, notwithstanding the ongoing difficulty with recruitment and retention of staff and doctors, relates to the management and prevention of workplace bullying and harassment. Such behaviours, in addition to the toll that they have on the individuals involved, impact patients and therefore the standard of care provided to them. There is the potential for harm to patients who are, essentially, innocent bystanders with regards the interactions between staff. Whilst this does not reduce or diminish the impact on those directly involved in such conflicts, as 'innocents', patients are completely unable to influence, respond to, or modify the impact of such behaviour on their clinical outcomes.

Behavioural incidents create significant harm in healthcare and, in particular, can have a significant impact of staff being made to feel intimidated in critical clinical situations. If a senior doctor's behaviour offends or intimidates a nurse in the theatres, that nurse may be impacted to the degree of not being able to speak up for safety in circumstances where patient safety was potentially compromised.

The tone in the operating theatre, bedside, or indeed, in any clinical area, is set by the most senior clinician who is present. If they are either responsible for poor behaviour themselves, or appear to condone, tolerate, or ignore poor behaviour from others, then staff and clinicians are unlikely to freely act, respond, or escalate their concerns. Multiple examples exist of occassions where the 'tone' of accepted poor behaviours and culture within healthcare has led to poor patient outcomes.

HR has a key role in influencing the culture and behaviour of a healthcare organisation by:

1. Ensuring that orientation of staff and doctors to the organisation aligns with the values, and the cultural expectations of the organisation, and making it clear how behaviour that doesn't align with these values could lead to direct and indirect impacts on patient care.
2. Articulating the expectations of managers and leaders in setting the tone and managing incidents relating to inappropriate behaviour.
3. Analysing staff experience and feedback in general and, in particular, feedback that is focused specifically on the culture of safety across the organisation.
4. Educating staff on and in leading investigations into behavioural incidents.

The complexity of power dynamics with respect to medical and nursing professionals and between senior and junior clinicians is a particular issue in healthcare. The challenge for HR professionals in healthcare is that in investigating behavioural incidents, often the clinical circumstances can complicate the issues being investigated.

Clinical authority and responsibility can often be used by staff and doctors in such circumstances to 'explain' or 'justify' inappropriate behaviours. This complicates HR investigations where navigating the issues to a successful resolution is often extremely challenging.

HR teams need to develop expertise in understanding these challenges and to be able to work together with clinicians and managers to help establish a culture of patient safety as well as a culture of psychosocial safety for staff. Importantly, assisting with ensuring that all staff feel safe to escalate concerns and challenge senior persons when there is concern for patient safety is key to the role of HR executives. Arranging and conducting transparent, fair, and comprehensive investigations into behaviour and related incidents is also critical.

2.5.2 Chief Financial Officer (CFO)

The CFO's challenge for any business is apparent and significant. However, it is critical that the CFO also understands the key clinical governance drivers that impact the financials of the business.

For example, reducing labour costs may show savings on a financial statement; however, the consequent clinical governance impacts of having fewer staff or under-trained and under-experienced staff are often difficult to measure. If an adverse clinical or staff incident does occur because of such a financial decision, it is uncommon that the responsibility for these rests with the CFO. Similarly, failure to invest in replacing equipment, maintaining equipment to required standards, or using 'cheaper' alternatives in medical or clinical equipment that will result in poorer clinical outcomes, rarely affects those who often make such decisions.

Newer medications are usually more expensive than the 'older' medications they replace but are usually readily adopted by clinicians because of clear benefits to the patient. For example, new agents with less side effects, which are easier to administer and generally better tolerated by the patient, are inevitably more expensive. The finance team may raise concerns in these circumstances where it appears that the replacement costs of a medication may have noticeable financial impacts. In this type of scenario, the CFO will often ask the clinical executive to 'engage with the clinicians' and ask them to change their practice or to restrict their use of the newer medication so that the 'older medication' returns to use and the financial cost returns to 'normal'.

It is critical in these types of circumstances that the CFO and finance team understand the difficulty and inappropriateness of negotiating with clinicians where the outcome relate purely to 'cost savings' only, without any other tangible benefit to the clinicians or their patients. To engage clinicians in cost-saving measures then, it is imperative that the finance team understands the clinical governance impact of these issues. As an example, if the use of a particular medication results in an increase in hospital-acquired infections (HAIs), or a change in staff rosters appears directly related to an increase in clinical incidents, then the CFO and the finance team need to incorporate and consider these outcomes in their financial decision-making, i.e. the clinical governance impact needs to be measured and demonstrated in financial terms.

Similarly, when reviewing business cases, there needs to be consideration of any unintended consequences that may lead to an increase in clinical incidents. Acknowledging the financial costs of clinical incidents and putting a 'price' on them provides for a more balanced financial perspective to be taken.

The CFO should ask about the clinical governance impacts of financial decisions that are being considered, understand the impact of unintended clinical consequences, request support in engaging clinicians, involve clinicians when enacting cost-saving strategies, and seek clinician's advice on opportunities that may exist to make further improvements.

2.5.3 Chief Marketing and Communications Officer

When clinical governance incidents occur, the C-suite executive responsible for media, communications, and marketing is responsible for ensuring that the reputation of the organisation is not damaged and that any risk of damage is mitigated. There are several key issues that these teams must be aware of in the context of healthcare clinical governance within their roles:

1. Ensuring compliance with regulatory requirements in relation to advertising and marketing of clinical innovations.
2. Monitoring for social media complaints, incidents and potentially damaging commentary.
3. Managing the reputational consequences arising from clinical governance incidents.

This role needs to balance the understandable enthusiasm for promoting clinical innovation, which often relates to an individual or a small number of clinicians, with understanding the potential for unexpected consequences and risks of such innovations. To avoid such circumstances, the marketing/communications team should engage closely with the clinical executive, to ensure that appropriate clinical governance processes have been followed.

There are several notable examples where media teams have undertaken promotional activities in relation to specific clinicians and/or innovations embroiled in investigations in relation to clinical governance issues, which due to a lack of communication with the clinical executives, they, had not been aware of.

In responding to enquiries or providing commentary following clinical incidents, the media team's common approach is often to avoid open and transparent communication and to attempt to 'close down' further discussion as soon as possible. However, in these circumstances particularly, it's important to ensure and openly demonstrate that the values of the organisation are actually 'lived' and maintained, by ensuring the expressions of condolences, sympathy, and similar appropriate sincere comments are made authentically and without compromising legal obligations.

It is particularly important for clinicians and all parties involved, including the community at large, to 'see', and indeed for all parties involved, as well as the community at large, to 'see' a healthcare organisation respond in an authentic and empathetic manner. The unintended consequences of 'blunt' and 'templated' comments that appear to lack empathy by media teams can be very damaging to the organisation and can lead to distress for all those involved.

2.5.4 Legal Counsel

Health lawyers and their teams are critically positioned to have a significant impact on the clinical governance of healthcare systems. They have an important role in ensuring that medico-legal cases are managed appropriately, that the organisation's insurance policies are complied with, and where feasible, the premium payments for medical malpractice insurance are reduced, by demonstrating robust clinical governance systems and processes that are continuously improved. This team is well placed to support the tone of how an organisation responds to a clinical incident.

It is well established that providing an apology at the time of an incident does not compromise the medico-legal liability and management of a case that is associated with a clinical incident. The legal team has a crucial role in supporting clinicians with providing an apology to patients and families, and in guiding them with responding to the legal complexities involved. Similarly, when negotiating organisational insurance contracts, this team can promote the clinical governance systems and processes that are in place at the organisation by demonstrating to the insurers how the processes assist in preventing clinical incidents, in mitigating the risk and impact of an incident. Emphasising the clinical governance systems for clinical audit, mortality and morbidity reviews, doctor credentialing, and for clinical incident management when negotiating with the insurers, can often result in more favourable terms being reached.

The legal team also plays an important role in influencing the tone that is set through the various correspondence they have with patients, families, coronial courts, regulatory, and other similar agencies. Whilst legal teams need to maintain and adhere to legal/insurance compliance requirements, they must demonstrate empathy and use appropriate language in keeping with the values of the organisation, when practicing within healthcare settings. The legal team also hold other key responsibilities with regard to consent, privacy, and legislative/regulatory compliance with clinical governance standards.

2.5.5 Chief Information/Technology Officer

Healthcare IT teams are increasingly being challenged by the risk of privacy breaches and maintaining the security of IT systems. With electronic medical records now being routinely utilised throughout healthcare services, the patchy yet increasing introduction of artificial intelligence into healthcare systems, and the multiple, well-publicised security breaches of healthcare data systems, the role of the CTO and IT team in clinical governance is growing in significance.

The IT team, working closely with both the financial and clinical governance team, has an increasing role in clinical governance, particularly with respect to assisting these teams in analysing clinical and financial outcomes. These roles relate to:

1. Managing data privacy, storage, and security
2. Enabling the use of compatible and user-friendly platforms to display data trends in analysis
3. Securely transmitting relevant clinical information that ensures patients are not 'lost' in the system
4. Monitoring and combining data from different areas of the system and bringing them together for analysing trends, benchmarking, and comparisons.

2.5.6 Clinical Executive: Chief Medical Officer (CMO) and Chief Nursing Officer (CNO)

As outlined earlier, the clinical executive has clear and specific responsibility and accountability for clinical governance. These roles, however defined, lead in several areas, including in:

- Establishing clinical governance frameworks
- Determining key indicators to monitor
- Developing clinical governance strategies
- Prioritising clinical governance elements for implementation
- Clinician credentialing and scope of practice (SOP)
- Hospital accreditation
- Clinical incident management
- Clinical audit and review
- Mortality and morbidity review
- Risk management
- Education and training in safety, quality, and clinical governance
- Research in clinical governance
- Consumer engagement and participation
- Innovation in clinical governance
- Setting the tone of a highly reliability organisation (HRO)
- Building the culture of clinical governance and speaking up for safety
- Public reporting, benchmarking, and clinical data analysis

2.6 Organisational Structure

The overarching governing committee responsible for patient safety and clinical governance sets the agenda for the organisation. Through its meetings, it ensures that the appropriate indicators are identified and monitored, that relevant interrogation of this data is undertaken, and further detail and information is obtained as required.

This group ensures that relevant information such as key clinical governance learnings are distributed and shared throughout the organisation so that all those involved in the delivery of patient care have a good understanding of safety, clinical outcomes, and performance. They also ensure that patient incidents have been appropriately investigated, managed, and that the recommendations and actions arising from them have been effectively implemented.

As the overarching clinical governance committee needs to prepares and provides reports for the executive and board, they should meet regularly with the board members and executives to ensure that there is a shared understanding of the status and potential risks that exist for patient safety.

Guided by the organisation's safety and quality plan, this committee should establish subcommittees for different areas of patient care as required. For example, if the organisation wishes to address Falls Prevention or Pressure Injury Prevention as areas of focus, then appropriate multidisciplinary subcommittees or working parties with expertise in these areas should be developed.

Participation in such sub-committees allows for deeper staff engagement and involvement in specific safety and quality aspects of patient care, and should also include patients and consumers at each level where possible. These groups should be tasked with reviewing current literature and best-practice models in the delivery of the particular patient safety focus area, adopt and implement best practices that are relevant to the organisation, and subsequently monitor and report on their effectiveness and performance. These committees and working parties can deep-dive into the data that is available to elicit a thorough understanding of which indicators are demonstrating unwarranted variations and to identify specific areas for improvement where relevant.

To ensure that all relevant key stakeholders are involved in the composition of such groups, it is important that these committees and working parties are multidisciplinary and involve non-clinical team members who may be critical in contributing to the provision of safe patient care. For example, membership of staff from IT services and other administrative support services who can assist clinicians in the development and rollout of new programs in patient safety must not be overlooked.

It is usually at this sub-committee level where quality improvement projects are considered and business cases for such projects are developed for approval by the overarching committee and/or executive. Sub-committees are also well placed to advise on the education and training programs, innovative areas of practice being considered, and any research opportunities if available.

Sub-committees can support the development of smaller working parties and teams to undertake specific projects and lead the implementation of improvements on the ground, as needed. They can also work directly with clinicians to facilitate consistency in service delivery, particularly in ensuring consistent compliance with policy and procedures that impact patients.

As an example, a committee working on surgical safety as a priority can create teams of clinicians to look at different aspects of ensuring surgical safety in practice. This group should ideally also include admissions staff, pre-theatre staff, anaesthetics staff, and nursing staff, in addition to surgeons. A key challenge for organisations continues to be the effective engagement and involvement of medical practitioners in patient safety initiatives.

The executive responsible for clinical governance will usually have a team of staff reporting to them whose roles and responsibilities relate to ensuring that the clinical governance standards across the organisation are being upheld and that the performance of the organisation is as expected. Whilst it is the responsibility of everyone to ensure clinical governance and patient safety are at the forefront of clinical practice, the clinical governance team, however named, holds specific responsibility to provide specialist advice and support for clinical governance to all areas across the facility.

Ensuring hospital-wide accreditation and organisational compliance with standards is usually overseen at a jurisdiction, government, or an external group level. Whilst demonstrating compliance with accreditation standards in a hospital is a requirement for all clinicians, the clinical governance team will usually play a key leadership role in how the accreditation standards are complied with prior to and during accreditation review periods.

The clinical governance team will also usually be involved in significant clinical incident investigations and their management, including the development of reports for executives and the board, monitoring of the quality indicators and undertaking benchmarking activities.

2.7 Monitoring and Reporting

Whilst an organisation's clinical governance team, executive, and board will usually discuss and debate clinical indicators, engaging staff and doctors in these discussions in ensuring that patient safety is regarded as everyone's business is often challenging. A simple yet effective way to approach this is to directly ask them for their comments specifically with regard to which key indicators they believe should be monitored that reflects the day-to-day quality of care, as well as any indicators that can be monitored to show improvements in quality of care.

Engaging staff to identify quality indicators in this manner will assist in strengthening their continued involvement in assessing their own clinical practices' impact on the indicators, as well as close involvement in mitigating poor outcomes, and improving the outcome for patients. When engaging with staff regarding indicators, it is important to emphasise that they focus on the clinical indicators that they themselves may have an impact on, for which they can directly influenced improvements. It's also helpful to ask them to identify practices that they may know exists within different areas of the organisation or elsewhere, which they may wish to adopt.

In terms of determining the final suite of quality indicators, it's important to ensure that they are able to capture not just clinical outcomes but also the quality of care and the patient experience.

To maintain genuine engagement with staff and reinforce the importance of patient safety, indicators should be prepared for publication and wider communication. This should be undertaken with recognition that the collection and interpretation of such indicators are resource-intensive and complex.

Ensuring that the resources required for the collection of data are available for the teams undertaking this work, is a key function of leadership in this space. Providing the adequate training and education required to understand how to interpret this data, how to translate and how to adapt the data to inform useful improvement programs is clearly important.

In terms of patient experience and patient-reported outcome measures (PREMS and PROMs), the organisation, from a leadership perspective, should commit to ongoing patient experience surveys. Patients experience surveys traditionally have been done following discharge of patients from a service; however, increasingly, contemporaneous patient experience, i.e. whilst patients are in hospital, is being gathered.

Having an active program of reviewing, measuring, and responding to complaints and acknowledging compliments is a key component of understanding the service and patient experience. Involving patient representatives in leadership committees means that leaders are emphasising the importance of patient engagement and, therefore, are reflecting this expectation throughout the organisation.

Leaders should ensure that staff are able to provide feedback directly with regard to the safety and quality of care. This can be achieved via staff and doctor satisfaction surveys, and targeted surveying initiatives, to ask questions specifically about the culture of patient safety within the organisation.

A commitment must be made that the feedback from staff to such surveys will be considered, accepted, and that the actions the organisation will undertake in response are communicated to staff.

This ensures that staff will be involved in communicating areas of improvement and participating in working through action plans to achieve improvements in outcomes for patients. Leaders should ensure there is an environment available for continuous learning with regard to safety and quality of care so that staff have sufficient time and professional development opportunities to improve their knowledge in this space.

2.8 Engaging Clinicians

Engagement with clinicians through clinical review and incident management can be a very successful strategy. Working with clinicians as part of the open disclosure process, speaking with the family and other authorities of the incident, and supporting clinicians through this process can establish good working relationships between the clinicians and healthcare leaders.

Involving clinicians in the analysis of cases and asking them what improvements might be possible, allows them to come up with the solutions themselves, which is more likely to lead to the successful implementation of those improvements.

Communicating the improvements to all clinicians, including those who may not have been involved in the case, allows for shared and collective learning. Informing clinicians of these system improvements can increase their engagement with the organisation.

The clinicians who are involved in the case can in fact become leaders of change, reflecting and recognising the changes and improvements they have made to the organisation.

Both administrative and clinician leaders are well placed to actively demonstrate and encourage a culture of patient-centric clinical incident management.

Patient-centric clinical incident management (PCCIM) involves having a robust process for the incident reporting, review and analysis, including an outcome-based improvement program from the analysis undertaken.

The difference to the 'standard approach' of incident management is that PCCIM is undertaken *with* the patient involved throughout the entire process, with the management of the case being considered from *their* perspective. Central to this approach is seeing the case 'through the lens of the patient' whilst keeping a focus on preventing repeats of the incident and improving systems to enhance outcomes.

As part of incident management, leaders should ensure that there is a 'just' culture in place with avoidance of blame and a commitment to adopt improvement programs for implementation following incident review.

PCCIM involves interdisciplinary case discussions, which its membership should reflect, and ensuring independence within the review process, with the use of experts or specialists in the relevant area who are external to the facility or service, if required.

Leaders should ensure that learnings, actions, and recommendations from an incident are shared across the organisation to avoid the scenario where an incident at one hospital site is then repeated elsewhere in the health service or system, due to a failure to implement shared learnings.

Leaders can challenge themselves to see if they are setting the right tone for PCCIM, and for patient safety and clinical governance in general within the organisation, by asking the following questions:

1. Does our approach to incident management align with the values and purpose of the organisation?
2. Are there clear roles and responsibilities for all staff involved with regard to patient safety?
3. Is the leadership clearly accountable for clinical performance and quality of care?
4. In terms of incident management, is there a clear structure and membership composition of committees with clear reporting and analysis of data processes in place?

In providing for a culture of PCCIM, leaders need to set the tone with regard to the importance of open disclosure within the organisation. Leaders should make a conscious decision to ensure the implementation of 'open disclosure' is a key component of the process, and that it is embedded in all incident management cases, regardless of the degree of severity of the incident.

Leaders' commitment to PCCIM is an excellent approach to effective and authentic clinician engagement, as clinicians by their nature are attracted to this concept, because it strongly aligns with their clinical practice.

Open disclosure should be viewed by the organisation as an opportunity to ensure that when a patient has suffered harm, there is a commitment to acknowledging that harm, apologising, investigating how the harm occurred, and providing a commitment to preventing it from reoccurring.

Engagement strategies for healthcare leaders, particularly in relation to clinicians, involve listening to their concerns before making additional requests of them.

Even in terms of financial performance, clinicians can provide a range of proposals where financial performance can be improved and, particularly, where cost savings can be found. Involving them in the process of reviewing and improving financial performance can be a very successful engagement strategy.

Clinicians also respond better to accurate data and evidence. Providing the data and evidence of the outcomes of clinical care and other aspects of performance of the organisation and asking them for their interpretation and suggestions for improvement is also an extremely important and valuable engagement strategy.

Clinician leadership and engagement is an essential element of high-performing healthcare systems and can contribute significantly to many improvements across quality indicators. Importantly, doctor participation in hospital governance can lead to improved quality and safety. Whilst having clinical leaders at the apex of the organisation is very important, leadership by clinicians should occur at all levels throughout the system.

True engagement with clinicians requires trust to be developed between clinicians and the leaders of the organisation. This can be achieved by establishing a culture of willingness to share relevant data, by creating a shared vision, and by ensuring open communication and dialogue. There is accumulating evidence that successful collaboration between clinicians and leaders of an organisation results in improved care and clinical outcomes.

2.9 Engaging Doctors

Doctor and physician engagement is complicated and is often seen as the most difficult part of clinician engagement. Doctor engagement does not happen on its own, and organisations must use diverse strategies and initiatives to strengthen doctor engagement and leadership in healthcare.

Understanding and addressing the underlying characteristics of how doctors behave and act, assists leaders with genuine doctor engagement. For doctors to be engaged, they must feel that they have some influence in important decision-making. Doctors must feel they are involved in, for example, purchasing capital equipment, implementing new clinical services, and framing the strategy of the organisation.

It is difficult to engage with doctors who have busy clinical practices, and many doctors do not wish to undertake administrative roles. Where possible, doctors should be compensated for their work in 'administration'. They should also be encouraged, and given an opportunity, to develop their leadership skills. This is particularly the case when doctors are asked to engage and lead in clinical governance.

It is common for leaders to speak to a small group of doctors whom they 'trust' to advise them on issues and get the 'doctor view'. However, this does not necessarily mean that such 'trusted doctors' are in fact reflective of how all doctors may want to engaged or how they, indeed, 'think'. As invaluable as it is to speak to those who are trusted supporters, it is also important to go to those who are dissenters for their views, and prior to doing so, to understand the likely arguments they will make in terms of their level of complaint or dissatisfaction.

Before meeting with doctors, it is important for leaders to note that they will generally be meeting with them in their workplace and therefore arrange to meet after the doctor's clinical duties are completed. It is valuable for leaders to understand where possible, the doctors' sentiments on a particular topic prior to meeting with them.

There are often 'opinion leaders' in doctor groups, and it is important to have an understanding of who these are in the organisation. Likewise, doctors greatly value evidence and data accuracy, and prior to presenting any data to them, it is essential to ensure it is as accurate as possible; otherwise, it is likely to lead to failed engagement.

In healthcare, but in medicine in particular, there are both horizontal and vertical lines of authority, and understanding how this authority aligns within an organisation is key to engaging medical staff by healthcare leaders.

Doctors cannot just be engaged in safety and quality; they must also lead in this space, as they set the tone of how patient safety is undertaken in the hospital. An example of this is an operating theatre where doctors are not only key to patient safety but need to demonstrate clinical leadership, for example in conducting time-out in relation to surgical safety checklists. Doctors, as clinicians, are interested in patient stories, and the use of patient stories as part of the engagement process can be very successful. Leaders who engage doctors and doctor groups in clinical governance within their system will generally see improved clinical outcomes and an improved culture of patient safety.

2.10 Case Study 1: Clinical Governance Leadership

The Chief Medical Officer (CMO) of an organisation attends the orientation of all new staff members each month to introduce himself and welcome the new starters to the organisation. As part of the welcome, the CMO describes five ways that he undertakes his work at the organisation, keeping patient safety and clinical governance at the forefront of everything he does.

He welcomes the new staff members to consider these five elements and how they should be incorporated into how they work as they join the organisation.

1. The CMO describes the importance to him of hand hygiene, and how when he enters each clinical area and every patient room, he washes his hands prior to entering and on leaving. He carries on his keyring an attachment that opens the hand hygiene stations throughout the organisation. He states that it is not uncommon to find the hand hygiene pumps empty or not functioning. Therefore, by carrying a key, he is able to open the station and arrange a replacement hand sanitiser bottle. He describes having done so when a high-level politician entered the hospital, where otherwise there would've been a delay and unnecessary embarrassment for the organisation. The CMO reveals that he has carried the same key over the entire time he has been at the organisation and says that by demonstrating that he himself is not above replacing the sanitiser bottle or knowing how to do so himself reflects the importance of actually practicing hand hygiene. He welcomes all new staff to 'call out' if they ever see him entering or leaving a patient area without washing his hands. He says they are endorsed to approach him directly and, if they witness he hasn't washed his hands and the staff member is correct, he will publicly thank them for pointing out this error.

   Whilst hand hygiene is clearly important, the CMO then explains that this practice is not just a demonstration of hand hygiene, but a personal commitment to patient safety, and how everything we do as health leaders is centred on living the values of clinical governance, patient safety, and the quality of care provided at all times. He asks his new colleagues to adopt a similar practice of authenticity during their time at the organisation.

2. The CMO describes another important aspect of how he operates within the hospital. Each day, on passing a colleague in the corridor, he ensures both eye and verbal contact with staff. A simple good morning and an acknowledgement of the person, by name if he is familiar with them each time he passes them in corridors or workspaces. He says the importance of this is that it demonstrates the respect we must hold for each other and the critical roles that everyone plays in providing patient services. Although he admits he won't be able to recall the name of all staff members directly, he encourages them to use his name if they can remember, and if not, to simply acknowledge. This simple behaviour of showing respect for each other is an important part of setting the tone of a hospital culture.
3. If the CMO sees any waste around the hospital, such as pieces of paper on the floor, he disposes of it using gloves or some other protective device, and then washes his hands. He encourages others to do this as well with the rationale being that this demonstrates respect for the organisation and the facility that we work in, as this is an important part of the provision of safe care. When patients and their families see that the organisation and the staff have respect for where they work, even the simple measure of ensuring that the hospital is clean and void of waste, can send a strong message.
4. Lastly he speaks of the importance of demonstrating respect for patients, visitors, families, and other members of the community within the organisation. He states that it is not uncommon in healthcare to see that people visiting a facility are often 'lost' as they try to navigate their way through. Hospitals are confusing to get around, and whilst visiting a hospital the level of anxiety that visitors and family members often have for the care and wellbeing status of their loved one, can be exacerbated. When the CMO sees a person who may look lost, as invariably they are, he approaches them and asks how he may help them. This simple kindness almost always helps to alleviate their immediate concern by assisting them to find where they need to go, by either taking them there directly or obtaining the assistance of a staff member who can do so. This demonstrative act provides confidence to family and visitors that this organisation actually does care, and that they can trust that the staff show genuine empathy and compassion.
5. The CMO states that once a person has entered the facility, even if they are yet to go to the clinical area for receiving treatment, they should be considered a 'patient'. He encourages all staff members that if they see patients in the facility, such as in waiting rooms, preparing to go to surgery, or preparing for admission, where those individuals may seem distressed, in pain, cold, or in discomfort, to approach the patient and ask if there is anything they can do to assist. Even a simple measure of obtaining a warm blanket for a person waiting in a cold waiting room can go a long way to alleviate anxiety and provide encouragement and confidence in the organisation. If a staff member is not a clinician and feels they are out of their depth with regard to a patient, they are advised to seek assistance from the closest clinical area or raise the concern directly with their manager. However, accepting that patients and good clinical governance are everyone's

responsibility, sets the tone that patient safety and quality care start as soon as the patient enters the facility.

The CMO details a final practical element in his welcome for clinicians to the organisation, via the example of the Medical Emergency Response Teams (MERT). He explains that the tone set by MERT starts with the leader of the team when they arrive at the clinical situation for which their assistance has been called. The CMO explains the difference between the following two initial responses when called:

1. Why did you call for emergency help? versus
2. I am from the medical emergency team. How can I help you?

In the first scenario, the tone immediately positions the person who called for help having to 'justify' and 'explain' their rationale for calling for assistance. A junior staff member, or one that lacks confidence in their clinical acumen, can be set back at this point. They can then become anxious and nervous about calling the emergency response team in future for fear of being seen to potentially waste the time of senior clinicians. Indeed, the experience of having to explain oneself and answer numerous questions as to the 'why' such a call for help was needed can lead that individual to not call for assistance in the future in a timely manner.

Alternatively, introducing yourself as a member of the emergency response team and asking, 'how can I help?' sets a very different tone—one of collaboration, cooperation, and assistance. Instead of challenging the individual, this approach demonstrates that 'we are all here working together' to help this patient. The importance of senior clinicians working with junior staff, particularly in the early stages of their careers and assisting them in this manner as a junior officer starts, is extremely important for ensuring patient safety. The experiences that junior clinicians have in terms of interacting with senior staff can have long-term impacts on their clinical practice, sense of confidence, and how they themselves then go on to interact with other clinicians.

Further Reading

Dye, Carson F. Leadership in Healthcare. Essential values and skills. Third edition. 2017.
Cashman, K. Leadership from the Inside out: Becoming a Leader for Life, 2nd Ed. 2008.
Kouzes, J.M and Posner, B.X. The Leadership challenge: How to make extraordinary things happen in organisations. 5th Ed. 2012.
Hughes, R.L, Ginnett, R.G and Curphy, G.J. Leadership: Enhancing the lessons of experience. 8th Ed. 2015.
Kotter, J. What Leaders really do. Harvard Business review. Dec 2001.
Lee, F. If Disney ran your hospital: 9 and half things you would do differently. 2012.
Jennings K and Stahl-Wert J. The Service Leader: Five powerful actions that will transform you team, your business and your community. 2003.
Spurgeon P, Clark J. Medical leadership: the key to medical engagement and effective organisations. 2nd ed. London: Radcliffe Publishing; 2017.
Spurgeon PC, Long PW, Powell J, Lovegrove M. Clinical leadership a practical guide for tutors, trainees and practitioners. London: BPP Media; 2015.
Pickuth D. Healthcare Executives: the essentials for excellent in leadership and management. 2018.

3 Clinical Governance Committee Structures

Implementing a program of clinical governance and building a culture of safety and quality is dependent on both formal and informal organisational structures. This includes working parties, teams, and structured meetings.

The purpose of these meetings is to drive improvement and build a culture of patient safety. In addition, there is the opportunity to share learnings, review outcomes and data, and consider the implications of changes to policies, procedures, guidelines, and other developments in the safety and quality space.

At the apex of the structure sits typically the clinical governance committee (or board). This body holds the ultimate responsibility for the organisation's clinical governance framework. Its primary duties include:

Strategic Oversight: Developing and implementing the overall clinical governance strategy, aligning it with the organisation's wider strategic goals.

Policy Approval: Reviewing and approving policies related to clinical practice, risk management, and patient safety.

Performance Monitoring: Regularly reviewing key performance indicators (KPIs) related to clinical effectiveness, patient experience, and safety.

Accountability: Ensuring appropriate accountability for the delivery of high-quality care throughout the organisation.

Resource Allocation: Advocating for and overseeing the allocation of resources needed to support quality improvement initiatives.

Risk Management Oversight: Overseeing the organisation's risk register, focusing on clinical risk identification, mitigation, and regular review.

The clinical governance committee should consist of senior leaders from various disciplines, such as medical, nursing, allied health, and executive management, to ensure diverse perspectives. It is imperative that this committee has clear reporting lines to the executive leadership and the organisation's governing body.

© The Author(s), under exclusive license to Springer Nature Singapore Pte Ltd. 2026
L. Prado, S. Chandrasiri, *The Practice of Clinical Governance*,
https://doi.org/10.1007/978-981-19-7896-8_3

To effectively manage the various aspects of clinical governance, the main committee usually delegates tasks to subcommittees. These subcommittees provide a focused approach to specific areas and often report back to the main clinical governance committee with recommendations and updates. Common subcommittees include:

Clinical Audit Committee: Focuses on the systematic evaluation of clinical practice against defined criteria and standards. They oversee the audit process, review findings, and develop action plans to address identified deficiencies. Activities include prioritising areas for clinical audit, overseeing data collection and analysis, and monitoring the implementation of improvements based on audit findings.

Patient Safety Committee: Dedicated to improving patient safety and reducing adverse events. They are responsible for analysing incident reports and identifying trends, developing and implementing patient safety initiatives, promoting a culture of safety and open reporting, and overseeing the implementation of root cause analysis (RCA) for serious incidents.

Risk Management Committee: Focuses on identifying, assessing, and mitigating clinical risks. Their activities include maintaining the organisation's risk register, developing and reviewing risk management policies and procedures, and providing advice on risk reduction strategies and appropriate use of risk management methodology.

Mortality and Morbidity Committee: Reviews cases of patient mortality and significant morbidity to identify lessons learned and opportunities for improvement. It focuses on reviewing and analysing cases to understand causes of adverse events, identifying systemic issues that contribute to poor patient outcomes, and recommending changes to practice preventing future incidents.

Medicines Management Committee (or Pharmacy and Therapeutics Committee): Responsible for overseeing the safe and effective use of medications. Their duties include developing and implementing prescribed guidelines, monitoring medication usage, and identifying potential adverse drug reactions, ensuring the availability and appropriate management of pharmaceuticals, focusing on clinical effectiveness and cost efficiency regarding medicines.

Infection Prevention and Control Committee: Focuses on preventing and controlling healthcare-associated infections. Key activities involve developing and implementing infection control policies and procedures, monitoring infection rates and identifying areas for improvement, and providing education and training on infection control practices. Other committee compositions are discussed below.

It is the responsibility of clinical leaders to set the 'tone' of staff engagement in safety and quality. Therefore, such leaders need to support the establishment of formal committee structures and at the same time encourage informal meetings of staff, where safety and quality are the focus of their agendas.

At the interface between the patient and clinician is where the first informal 'meeting' on safety and quality often takes place. Clinicians need to engage with patients and their families frequently in elements of safety and quality that relate to their care. Examples include discussion on falls prevention and medication safety, and how the patient and their family can participate in creating a safe environment by employing preventive actions that can 'keep themselves safe'.

Another area is the inclusion of the patient in the clinical handover process, which is done 'in the room or at the bedside', allowing the patient to be actively involved in their care, ask pertinent questions, and clarify any misconceptions and concerns.

In complex clinical circumstances, multidisciplinary team (MDT) clinical conferences, including all those involved in the patient care, are vitally important to ensure all clinicians are on the same page with regards to the treatment plan. This form of communication avoids errors, e.g. all outstanding results can be reviewed by the entire team, and all forms of clinical options can be considered.

These meetings are of two general types: The first relates to MDT meetings, where the purpose is to ensure that the most appropriate clinical course of action is determined with a focus on known best practice and 'gold standard' treatments. Examples include the management of cancers, where such meetings between individual specialists from each clinical discipline in coordinating the treatment plan, including surgical, radiation, chemotherapy, and immune therapy options. Such meetings allow for clarity in the follow-through of the plan, collection of clinical data, and post-treatment outcomes.

The second form of MDT relates to case conferencing with discussion of complex care issues relating to the physical, psychological, and emotional care of the patient, and the impact on family and other caregivers. Ideally, these conferences should include community/primary health care providers who are also involved in the patient's care.

In addition, the patient and family should be actively involved in these case conferences, so that the discussions and recommendations made are practical and implementable. These case conferences are key to the strength of clinical governance within the organisation as they take a patient-centric approach where the quality and safety of care are paramount and front of mind. When discussed between all clinicians, it assures that before decisions are made, there is a comprehensive conversation of all known facts and variables and risks, and all those involved in the care path are on the same page. This avoids error, misunderstanding, and potential for confusion.

Following on from the bedside clinical handover, shift and roster changes are another key opportunity for practical clinical governance to be actioned.

Team leaders in these situations set the tone of 'centering on the patients' whose care they are responsible with the other staff and team members. These 'informal' meetings are often identified as the 'first' missed opportunity in the event of clinical error, as most of these meetings are led by and composed of junior staff members and can often include locum/agency staff and others who may not be as familiar with the policies, procedures, and clinical guidelines of the organisation. Therefore, whilst considered 'informal', these meetings are in fact key to ensuring the safety and quality of patient care.

Examples of the discussion that occurs at such meetings often include:

- Current clinical states of each patient.
- Clinical concerns regarding potential changes in state.
- Follow-up of outstanding investigations and results.
- Medications to be dispensed.
- Patients who are at high risk for falls, sepsis, delirium, and other incidents.
- Social and psychological aspects of the patient's care.

These meetings also provide an opportunity to review any recent changes to policies and any focus areas that the team considers important, such as a focus on falls prevention or medication safety. Although informal, these meetings should have notes taken and follow a well-developed checklist or other proforma to ensure adequate effectiveness.

Within clinical or other patient care teams, there should be regular formal meetings where safety and quality are specific agenda items. If teams are well-resourced, there may be a dedicated safety and quality team member. However, if this is not the case, it is recommended that if the leaders themselves take on responsibility for the safety and quality portfolio, or another, preferably senior team member, take on the portfolio.

It is crucial that the safety and quality components at these meetings include:

- Recent clinical incidents within the team.
- Status of any ongoing clinical investigations.
- New policy, procedures, or guidelines.
- Local areas of concern for the team, e.g. medication safety.
- Team and unit processes that have been developed to prevent patient harm.
- Team clinical data such as patient experience, falls, pressure ulcers, and medication incidents that are discussed and evaluated.

The team meetings are the basis of the clinical governance culture within a healthcare organisation. Senior leaders should take the opportunity to 'round' at these meetings to encourage the dialogue that takes place and demonstrate their commitment to the safety and quality of patient care.

At the hospital or 'system' level, there are a range of cultures and meetings that are essential to the practical implementation of the clinical governance framework. Regardless of the specific structure a hospital determines to have in place, it is essential that there is clarity within the Committee Terms of Reference (TOR) as to:

- Scope of committee responsibility.
- Decision-making accountability and responsibility.
- To whom the committee reports.
- Ensuring that the committee has broad representation of clinicians, other key staff, and consumers/patients.

- Use of data, reports, and other clinical information that can assist the committee with their deliberations.
  Committees should consider the following:

1. Overarching clinical governance and safety and quality topics:
   (a) Policy and procedures
   (b) Clinical guidelines
   (c) Patient experience data
   (d) Risk management protocols
   (e) Clinical incidents review
   (f) Clinical outcome data
   (g) Horizon scanning of changes in the safety and quality environment, such as emerging trends and benchmarking
   (h) Opportunities for education, training, professional development, and research in clinical governance

2. Committees should focus on specific clinical risk areas, e.g.:
   (a) Infection prevention control
   (b) Falls
   (c) Medication safety
   (d) VTE (venous thromboembolism) prophylaxis

3. Committees should focus on programs to assure safety and quality, e.g.:
   (a) Patient experience surveys
   (b) Antimicrobial stewardship
   (c) Clinical incident review process
   (d) Mortality and morbidity meetings
   (e) Clinical audits programme and contribution to registry data
   (f) Surgical safety process

4. There is also a range of committees that bring together teams across the hospital organisation. Such committees include:
   - Policy and procedure committee e.g. high-risk medication prescribing and dispensing
   - Clinical guidelines committee e.g. antimicrobial stewardship
   - Clinical performance and practice improvement committee e.g. prevention of central line infections
   - Clinical outcome data committee e.g. falls prevention committee
   - Digital health and IT committee e.g. electronic medication management

Collaboration between teams/departments is critical for an organisation to embed the safety and quality culture and to align teams in the clinical governance space.

Such examples include:

(a) Supply/procurement working with safety and quality to ensure safety recalls and product warnings are actioned. This also allows clinicians to be engaged when new contracts are negotiated, tenders announced, and to hold discussions regarding new clinical equipment and supplies to ensure appropriate consultations take place.
(b) Clinical coding working with safety and quality to ensure that clinical outcomes, e.g. hospital-acquired complications, are coded correctly and that reports can be obtained to allow cross-referencing with clinical outcome data. This enables review of individual clinician performance, determining rates of incidents, facilitating benchmarking, reporting to regulatory authorities, and contributing to clinical registries and other external bodies and agencies.
(c) Digital/eHealth and IT working with safety and quality teams: Most IT applications throughout healthcare organisations will have an impact on the safety and quality agenda. The most obvious is the electronic medical record, where close collaboration between the clinical and IT teams (often facilitated by clinical IT experts) is critical. Such committees are also important for the successful implementation of new IT platforms, equipment, and other IT programs such as:

    - Clinical monitoring equipment
    - Telemetry equipment and smart devices
    - Data security and privacy breaches
    - Patient portals for admissions and clinical information
    - eHealth databases such as medication dispensing
    - Interconnection between platforms and programmes, e.g. monitoring and anaesthetic equipment linking to the EMR

(d) Finance and funding: These teams work with safety and quality staff on areas such as value-based healthcare (VBHC), contracting, pay for performance/outcomes, determining the cost of hospital-acquired complications, purchase of clinical equipment and other contracts, expenditure, and savings related to safety and quality.
(e) Biomed/infrastructure: These teams work with safety and quality staff to consider, for example infection control impact with regards to infrastructure changes/renovations, and the role of biomed in commissioning new clinical equipment, e.g. smart medication pumps.
(f) Legal services: These teams, which may be in-house or outsourced models, work closely with safety and quality teams in managing medico-legal claims, complaints, and clinical incidents.
(g) HR and education/training teams work closely with safety and quality teams to ensure the recruitment and retention of clinicians who are appropriately qualified, trained, and experienced and who are capable of working at the 'top of their licence/scope'.
(h) Risk and audit: The safety and quality team works with the risk and audit team to assess clinical risks as part of the group enterprise risk strategy and risk register and determine methods of mitigating and managing clinical risk. This has

a significant impact on how the risk of patient harm is managed and how well controls are working.

(i) Strategy: The safety and quality team works with the strategy team on the horizon scanning of new clinical services to ensure that safety and quality considerations are part of the strategic plan. The safety and quality team can contribute greatly to the development of the clinical services plan.

(j) Clinical/medical advisory councils/committees (MACs): The safety and quality team work closely with MACs and similar committees to ensure that they are engaged in the safety and quality agenda to leverage the expertise and support of the clinicians.

3.1 Safety and Quality Forums

Hospitals should consider establishing a forum, council, or senate devoted to safety and quality. These forums provide an opportunity for:

- Presentations on safety and quality topics, emerging trends, research, and new initiatives in this space.
- Communicating the overarching direction of the organisation in safety and quality.
- Obtaining feedback on the safety and quality agenda and direction of the organisation.
- Assessing the safety and quality culture.
- Clarifying practicalities of policies and procedures.
- Identifying areas of improvement to focus on.

Membership should be broad and include both clinical and non-clinical/support leaders and community/consumer representation.

3.2 Specialty Medical Craft Groups

It is important that clinicians working within the same clinical area come together regularly to discuss the standards of care provided, review clinical outcome data, consider morbidity and mortality reviews, consider clinical guidelines, review new technology and services, and undertake benchmarking activities. This can include medical speciality groups such as orthopaedic surgeons coming together to review clinical outcomes. Such groups are enhanced when other health professionals, e.g. nursing and allied health staff, are also members. There is also substantial benefit in teams who work together in the patient journey, e.g. cardiologists, cardiac surgeons, intensivists, and anaesthetists, collaboratively meeting to discuss cases and improvement opportunities in the complete patient care pathway (Fig. 3.1).

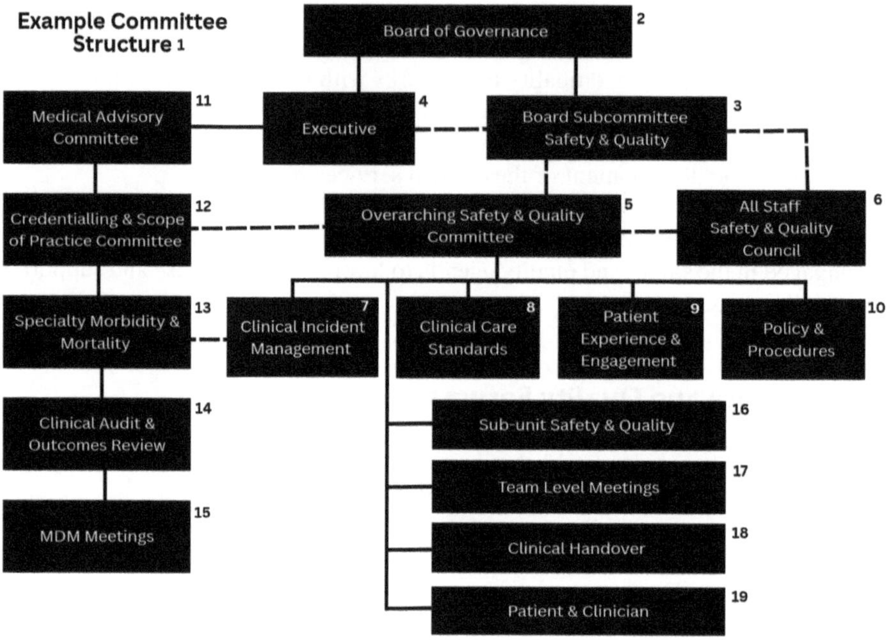

Fig. 3.1 Example clinical governance committee structure

4 Clinical Governance in Patient-Centric Incident Management

Clinical governance plays a crucial role in patient-centric incident management. It establishes a framework of accountability and continuous improvement, ensuring that patient safety is paramount. This framework promotes systematic reporting, thorough investigation, and proactive preventative strategies. By integrating data analysis from incidents into governance structures, healthcare organisations can identify systemic vulnerabilities and implement evidence-based solutions. The focus shifts from individual blame to a culture of learning and enhancement, ultimately fostering a safer environment for both patients and staff. Effective clinical governance provides the oversight and resources necessary to translate incident data into tangible improvements in patient care.

Despite the emphasis on clinical incident investigations as part of an effective incident management process, there still remains a number of important issues with how this is conducted in hospitals. Some of these issues include:

- Inconsistent governance arrangements.
- Inadequate team membership, including those who may lack sufficient training and expertise to manage or investigate the incident.
- Inconsistency regarding the determination as to how an incident is to be investigated.
- The standard of the quality of the investigation in terms of the depth and range of information reviewed, the line of enquiries undertaken, and the rigour of how the investigation is conducted.
- Often investigations are conducted thoroughly but the recommendations that come from the investigations lack meaningful impact and, often, relate to 'additional resources' for training, and changes to policies and procedures. More meaningful recommendations in terms of changing behaviours and improvement in delivery of care can be challenging.
- Implementation of recommendations and seeing that the recommendations have been implemented throughout the organisation, following up of the processes

© The Author(s), under exclusive license to Springer Nature Singapore Pte Ltd. 2026

L. Prado, S. Chandrasiri, *The Practice of Clinical Governance*,
https://doi.org/10.1007/978-981-19-7896-8_4

and monitoring the impact of the implementation of the recommendation, continue to prove challenging. Despite the best attempts of those involved, consistent failure to share learnings continues to be highlighted by organisations.

- Members of investigation teams often reflect they have not been provided feedback in terms of the investigation outcomes being implemented and how their involvement was, therefore, impactful across the organisation.
- Another fundamental problem with the current incident management approach to improving safety and quality is that, by its nature, it reflects on a 'case-by-case' clinical incident scenario. There are many examples where organisations continue to review the same 'type' of clinical incident, making 'ongoing' similar recommendations, and yet the implementation of the recommendations and change of practice do not occur.

A more contemporary framework of patient-centric incident management is one that is values-driven, patient- and family-focused, and empathic in nature. There is a focus on the language, tone, and content of incident management, requiring the agreement of the board and alignment with the medico-legal teams for it to be successful. Such an approach ensures group-wide consistency in terms of incident investigations and group-wide learning and sharing of implementations and recommendations.

4.1 Case Study 1: Outsourced Service Governance Failure

A 56-year-old gentleman was admitted for an elective vascular procedure to be performed late in the afternoon, and although a complicated procedure in itself, it was expected to proceed without significant issues.

However, after 2 hours of operating, there was a significant complication, and the patient suffered massive blood loss. This led to a period of clinical instability and required the patient to receive several interventions, including intravascular support, and further support for his kidney and respiratory functions.

At the end of the surgery, due to the patient's precarious clinical condition, he was transferred to the ICU for stabilisation. On arrival at ICU, his condition, although serious, was stabilised by the medical and nursing team, and over the next hours his condition remained stable.

In the early hours of the morning, unfortunately, he sustained a further bleed, and at this point his condition destabilised. The clinical team determined that an urgent return to theatre was required for stabilisation of his medical condition. Due to the nature of the blood loss, he had required a number of interventions, including support for his heart, lungs, and kidneys. Therefore, in arranging the transfer from the ICU to the operating theatre, the team prepared for the movement of these key pieces of clinical equipment to accompany the patient during the transfer to the operating theatre.

The operating theatre was one floor away, and therefore transport required the use of the nearby elevators. In preparing the patient, the operating team attended the ICU, and the surgeon and anaesthetist reviewed the patient and determined to accompany the patient to the theatre.

In addition to the operating team, an intensive care medical officer and external (contracted) technicians monitoring the equipment attached to the patient were to accompany the patient on transfer. The ICU Nurse was also prepared for transfer to monitor the patient's clinical observations.

The transfer commenced from the theatre to the elevator and initially progressed well. However, just prior to entering the elevator, one of the key pieces of vascular equipment failed, and it was at that point the clinical team realised the patient's circulatory system had suddenly become severely impacted.

The team reviewed the situation as quickly as possible and determined that the external technician (responsible for this equipment) appeared unfamiliar with how to rectify the situation and they felt that the equipment could not be immediately restarted during transfer. The team rapidly took the patient from the elevator through to the operating theatre, at which point the equipment was connected to the wall power supply and appeared to function normally.

The patient underwent surgery for a number of hours, and during the procedure, his condition stabilised. Following the operation, the patient was returned to the ICU. However, during the post-operative period, it became apparent that the patient had sustained a hypoxic brain injury as a result of the period of time that the circulatory support equipment had failed during transfer.

Although this was not identified initially, it was realised during attempts to wean the patient off the ventilator. Concerns had been raised during the patient's initial return to ICU that indeed complications such as hypoxia may have ensued during the transfer. This was raised by the clinical staff who attended the patient at that time, who were concerned that a vital piece of equipment had failed during transport.

Although the patient initially recovered from this urgent surgery, unfortunately his condition continued to deteriorate, and attempts to wean the patient off the ventilator failed, where it was determined that the patient had indeed suffered a significant hypoxic injury, from which recovery was unlikely.

Following discussions with the family, it was decided the patient would be managed in a palliative manner from that point, and subsequently passed away some days after the original surgery.

4.1.1 Standard Case Management

The intensive care team reviewed the patient's death as part of their usual mortality review process. The process identified that the patient had had an elective surgery late in the day for a serious condition. This meant that the patient returned to the ICU at a time when more junior medical staff were in attendance. However, due to the seriousness of the patient's condition, the senior consultants had arrived at the hospital to review the patient not long after admission, and this was deemed an appropriate response.

The investigation determined the following: The patient's clinical deterioration overnight had been rapidly identified and escalated appropriately, and the decision to return to theatre was deemed to be appropriate. The transfer team that had been established to take the patient to the operating theatre was experienced in transfers at this hospital, from ICU to theatre.

Although this patient required multiple pieces of equipment as part of the transfer to return to theatre, this was not unusual, as this was often the case with patients in ICU who had to return to theatre.

The transfer had occurred in the early hours of the morning, and this meant that few staff were available at the time of the transfer. It was noted in the review that the patient's clinical condition had deteriorated during transfer due to the failure of a piece of critical equipment. It was noted that this failure had been identified rapidly, that staff had noted and escalated that the equipment had failed, and as a result the patient's clinical condition had deteriorated.

The decision to continue to the theatre at this point rather than pause and either (1) Return to the ICU, or (2) Attempt to rectify the failed equipment during transport was debated at length. Due to the fact that the equipment failure had been recognised, but the team present was unable to rectify the situation rapidly, the decision to go to the operating theatre was deemed appropriate.

The operation itself and the management of the patient in the operating theatre and subsequently in ICU were deemed to be appropriate. The hypoxic brain injury was determined to be due to circulatory failure during the transfer, a situation that, once it had occurred, would not be seen to be resolvable.

The review team identified that there were some issues regarding the transfer. This included a transfer 'checklist' not having been in place, therefore it was considered appropriate to consider the adoption of a transfer 'checklist' prior to moving a patient from the ICU to the operating theatre. Due to the criticality of the equipment failure, the hospital's biomedical team was asked to immediately review the equipment to determine if the failure had been unpredictable or one that could have been mitigated.

Critical equipment failure was attributed as being the root cause of the patient's deterioration, and although tragic, was not predictable and would not have been able to be managed in any other manner at the time. The clinical team's response therefore had been appropriate whilst the circumstances were unfortunate, which then led to the patient's demise.

The quality and safety team reviewed the incident and determined that the clinical review had captured the most important clinical practice issues that had occurred. The clinical care provided had been appropriate, and the responses to the patient's condition had been appropriate.

The biomedical team advised that the equipment had failed due to a failure of the internal battery. The reason the equipment was able to be used once in the operating theatre was that the internal battery had been bypassed, and the wall power supply had been able to re-establish the equipment to normal function.

On further review of the equipment maintenance records, a number of further issues were identified. The equipment was not owned by the hospital but was on loan from a third-party provider, and the technician on duty at the time was provided by the third-party to monitor and maintain the equipment during transfer. As the equipment was on loan, the maintenance records of the hospital were incomplete and it was unclear as to how long it had been since the equipment had been serviced, and how long particularly it had been since the battery had been serviced or replaced.

The biomedical team enquired further and determined that the battery itself had been due for replacement at least 12 months prior to the incident. They confirmed that the equipment had not been serviced as required by the manufacturer's specifications.

The third-party providers were formally requested to review the equipment, who then confirmed that the battery had failed. They further confirmed that the battery had been due for service and indeed for replacement, and that neither had occurred.

The company provided information that in the event the equipment failed due to a lack of power, there was a manual override that could be used. The technician on duty had not experienced a situation requiring the use of the manual override nor felt adequately trained, and therefore felt unable to do so during the transfer.

The technician's decision to recommend immediate transfer to the operating theatre rather than attempt to use the manual override was deemed appropriate, as the time to theatre would appear to have only been a matter of minutes, whilst his lack of familiarity with the manual override may have resulted in a longer time to re-establish the equipment to its functioning state.

The company advised that further training and practical experience regarding the manual override would take place, that their policy and procedures for the management of equipment failure due to power supply would be remedied, and that they would comply and ensure the equipment would be maintained into the future appropriately, including battery replacement.

The safety and quality team were concerned with the response from the company and escalated this to the executive of the hospital. The hospital executive concluded they were unsatisfied with the processes in place with the company and provided a 'show cause' as to why the company would be allowed to continue to provide this clinical service to the hospital.

The safety and quality team, following the revelation as to the role of equipment failure and the causes, advised the family of the circumstances of the failure and that this likely contributed significantly to the patient's clinical deterioration. However, they explained that it was not possible to categorically confirm that the period of hypoxia was directly and solely related specifically to the equipment malfunction. The lack of clarity in this regard was thought to be due to the severity of clinical disease the two urgent operations and length of time spent in ICU all having the potential to contribute to the likelihood of developing hypoxic brain injury.

The monitoring of the patient during transfer however, did show a direct impact on the patient's circulatory support due to the loss of power. This was complicated by the fact that during this time the nursing staff were only able to record certain components of the monitoring as they had been focused on the emergency response to the deterioration of the patient and had not recorded all observations.

On enquiry, the electronic monitoring record of observations that should've been obtained during the transfer was informed as having not downloaded into the ICU IT system and therefore was now lost and not available for review. The patient's family were advised of the findings above. They were unsatisfied with the duration of the investigation, which had taken a matter of months, and the lack of communication from the investigation team in that time. The family further felt that the fact that equipment failure and maintenance issues had not been identified earlier and had not been disclosed to them in the first 24–48 hours, and therefore the response from the hospital was significantly lacking.

4.1.2 Patient-Centric Incident Management

When using the 'Patient-centric-incident Management' framework, there is a different approach to how an incident is managed. This includes a focus on the patient and family, and the prompt identification of 'immediate actions' that could be undertaken by the organisation to ensure no further harm occurs, as well as to prevent a repeat of the incident whilst the investigation is being undertaken. This same case will now be considered under the 'Patient-centric Incident Managment' approach.

The patient's clinical deterioration had been recognised during the transfer and was known by the operating team, ICU, and the supporting transfer staff in the early hours of the morning. Therefore, it was apparent there was no issue with regards the identification of the clinical deterioration.

In view of the criticality of the piece of equipment that failed, once this was identified that morning, the CMO held an Immediate Action Meeting (IAM), at which it was determined that all surgical procedures requiring its use would be either immediately suspended and patients transferred, or a replacement piece of equipment immediately sought across all facilities and sites within the hospital group. As a result of the IAM, no further procedures were undertaken until the biomedical team could confirm that the equipment was functioning normally as required and expected. An IAM is a meeting that is held as soon as possible following a serious incident that identifies on-going risks and 'needs' of the patient/family, staff and any immediately identified safety issues that can either be managed or at least mitigated until the formal investigation is completed. Done effectively it means that the hospital or organisation is not waiting for the report from an investigation some weeks or months later, to instigate actions which are clearly identifiable as an immediate risk at the time of the incident.

An urgent review of the equipment checking process in the ICU was undertaken. This included the processes for checking that there was an adequate power supply, and checking of the functioning of all battery-operated equipment in the ICU, operating theatres, and other critical areas. This process was then immediately implemented as an ongoing routine and regular check across the hospitals.

The IAM raised concerns with potential failures in governance regarding the management of equipment, recording of maintenance, and ensuring equipment resupply. Records for third-party contract management across the hospital group were reviewed and found to be inconsistent. As a result, it appeared that third-party providers were 'left to their own devices' with regards to the maintenance, repair, and replacement of key clinical equipment. The CMO therefore directed that an immediate review of these processes be undertaken and any and all other 'third-party' equipment be identified.

At the IAM, it was noted that the credentialing and scope of practice of technicians from third-party providers was another aspect that was found to be inconsistently applied. The experience and training of third-party technicians with regard to the management of equipment, particularly at times of critical failure, were also found to be inconsistent and inadequate.

A system for how the third-party providers communicated and provided assurance to the hospital of their staff having met all training and experience requirements, particularly in responding to situations of critical equipment failure, was also found to be absent.

This case highlights the importance of the following considerations by using an IAM approach within a Patient-centric Incident management framework:

1. Early escalation of a clinical incident that can have a significant impact not only for the individual patient involved, but also for other patients who may be in similar situations elsewhere at the hospital, and across other sites and facilities within a group of hospitals in the same system.
2. The governance systems involved in the use of clinical equipment provided by third-parties needs to robust and competent, as this is a common scenario in hospitals. Ensuring staff credentialing, monitoring of training, experience, and ongoing professional development, as well as the availability and access to those records by the hospital, is critical. The collaboration of third-party providers with hospital staff in team-based training, such as simulated scenarios on responding to critical incidents and crisis situations involving equipment failure, is required. Records of maintenance, supply, and repair need to be comprehensive, including when third parties are responsible for equipment. Regardless of the responsibility of another entity, the hospital needs to have appropriate governance regarding contract management and management of any piece of equipment that is residing within the hospital.
3. When equipment failure occurs, it is important that all other sites where the equipment may be in place are immediately notified of the equipment failure, that an immediate review of the equipment's performance can be undertaken, and that, if in doubt, the equipment is embargoed until confirmation has been received that it is functioning normally.
4. Equipment testing, particularly where batteries are involved, ensures that equipment is functioning normally on both internal and external power supplies. It's important that this testing occurs regularly, and is appropriately recorded. For equipment managed by third parties where their failure may impact on clinical care, the hospital teams also need to be familiar with the management of that particular equipment, including any override systems and any other responses that are possible, even if those are normally undertaken by a third-party technician.

5. Clinical Transfer Planning must be in place, as this is often found to have been inadequate following an incident. A 'checklist' for ensuring all equipment is functioning prior to undertaking a transfer must be conducted.
6. Finally, disclosure to the patient's family that a key piece of clinical equipment had failed did not occur as required by the hospital's policy on open disclosure. Delayed disclosure to the family resulted in significant stress and anger and resulted in the triggering of a difficult relationship with the hospital and the clinicians, which could have been avoided.

The clinician involved in the case was significantly impacted from a professional and personal perspective, as a key piece of clinical equipment failure had caused the patient harm and resulted in significant stress to all those involved whilst under his care. A major learning from this review was the understanding of the impact of such incidents on clinicians. Recognising and addressing the impact on clinicians is key with regard to their engagement with and adoption of future system and process improvements.

4.2 Case Study 2: Medical Device Failure

A 42-year-old woman was admitted as a day case for a routinely scheduled gynaecological procedure by an experienced specialist gynaecologist. The procedure required resection of the uterine lining, during which a specialised medical device was used to assist. This device was recently purchased by the hospital to replace an older model that had been in use for many years, with which the clinical staff had been very familiar with. As this version of the device was relatively new and the staff unfamiliar in its use, a representative of the manufacturer was present to assist. The device had been promoted as a major upgrade from what had been in use previously.

During the procedure, the patient's clinical condition suddenly deteriorated, and the patient arrested. Although initial resuscitation was successful, the patient subsequently died in the Intensive Care Unit. Whilst initially the cause of death was unclear, it was subsequently determined that an air embolism was to blame. In view of the seriousness of the case, a full clinical investigation was initiated. Whilst this was being undertaken, a second similar case occurred. The second case involved a different clinician and clinical team using an identical, but second similar device. This second incident occurred in another hospital that was owned by the healthcare group.

As the two cases occurred at two different facilities, they were linked within the healthcare group's clinical incident management system, alerting the central clinical governance team.

From the local investigations carried out at each of the two hospitals, it was noted that in the second case, although the patient survived, they too appeared to have suffered from an air embolism.

4.2.1 Standard Case Management

Each hospital's local clinical covernance team commenced their individual incident investigations, including ongoing open disclosure with the impacted (second) patient and the first patient's family respectively. Investigations included obtaining detailed reports from the clinicians involved, obtaining independent expert opinions, and reviewing medical practitioner credentialing, their scopes of practice, case volume, clinical outcomes, and specific experience in the procedure that was undertaken. The investigations concluded that the cause of the clinical deterioration due to the air embolism was unclear; however, it was likely due to equipment failure and/or practitioner technique. The following documents were obtained and steps undertaken as part of the two separate investigations:

- Medical reports from the gynaecologist, surgical assistant, and anaesthetist.
- Reports from the theatre suite nurse, scout nurse, and anaesthetic technician.
- Report from the code blue team.
- Reports from the intensive care unit team.
- Analysis of the two medical devices by the biomedical teams.
- Reviews completed by the clinical director of the unit, and the director of critical care, including consideration being given to the indications for the procedures, the procedure itself, and the reports provided by clinicians.
- Case reviews at the clinical audit meeting (morbidity/mortality).
- Review of the report from the coronial autopsy
- Review of the clinical case by an independent specialist gynaecologist.
- Review of each medical practitioner's scope of practice, case volume, and clinical outcomes.

The central clinical governance team remained concerned that two almost identical cases had occurred within weeks of each other, involving two different surgical teams, two devices of the same model and in two different surgical suites. A number of key issues of concern were particularly noted:

1. That there was little evidence of clinicians having had experience with using the newer model of the device, although both gynaecologists had extensive experience conducting the procedure using the older model. It was noted however, that representatives of the manufacturer were present in both cases.
2. That air embolism is a very uncommon cause of cardiac arrest in these circumstances, and the mechanism of the cause of embolism remained unclear.
3. That in both cases, the patient had no apparent predisposing medical conditions that could have contributed to the clinical risk.

4.2.2 Patient-Centric Incident Case Management

The case will now be considered using the Patient-Centric Incident management framework. In view of the two cases occurring over a short period of time and concerns noted, the central clinical governance team called for an IAM (Immediate Action Meeting) which enabled a number of additional steps to be undertaken as part of the investigation to better understand the circumstances that had occurred:

- Review of current clinical literature to determine whether any case reports of a similar nature had been published.
- Search of safety and quality alerts/updates and similar notices for evidence of similar case reports.
- Request to the manufacturer for information on any similar cases that may have been reported to them.
- Request for a mechanical review of the two devices to determine if any fault or failure of performance was evident, including a review of their previous services, testing, and maintenance needs.
- Request to the jurisdictional safety and quality entity for any information on any known similar clinical events.
- Request to the national medical regulatory body for any information on any known similar events occurring.
- Contact with other hospital sites at which this new piece of equipment was in use to determine if any other incidents had occurred.
- Contact with the specialist regulatory medical college for any information of similar cases.

As this information was compiled, under the direction of the Chief Medical Officer, the following actions took place:

- Health service-wide temporary moratorium on the use of all models of the medical device in question.
- Formal advisory to all clinicians on the moratorium and reasons for the initiation of the safety alert.
- Formal notification to the device manufacturer of the concerns.
- Formal notification to the jurisdictional safety body.
- Formal notification to the national regulation body.
- Formal notification to the specialist college.
- Formal notification to the chief medical officers of other hospitals where the equipment was in use, regarding the decision to place a temporary hold on the use of the device.

The CMO then commenced a comprehensive investigation of the clinical scenario including reproducing a theatre ‘set-up’ and the procedure undertaken, in the simulation centre. The simulation compared the use of the new device with that of the previous model and an alternative ‘set-up’ used by many other clinicians. The simulation identified significant concerns with how the new model functioned in comparison to the older model, including the presence of very different monitors and dials. The variance was such that clinicians were not aware of the need to undertake a different protocol in undertaking the procedure, and that there was a need to change how the equipment was monitored whilst it was being used.

Adopting a 'Patient-centric Incident management' approach in the investigation process highlights the importance of the following:

1. Ensuring that the clinical governance system in place at a health service are able to identify when similar/like clinical situations occur (even if at different sites and facilities), to enable a coordinated process. Such a centralised process ensures that system-wide issues can be more easily identified and silo investigations can be avoided.
2. The responsibility to provide early notifications of a concern regarding a procedure or medical device, in the interest of public safety.
3. Rapid escalation and notification of a significant clinical risk to the appropriate external professional bodies and regulatory services.
4. Relentless pursuit of in-depth investigation and analysis of the circumstances when faced with a confusing scenario where the sequence of events remains unclear.
5. Thorough understanding of the process involved in the introduction of a piece of clinical equipment into the organisation. The process for the introduction of a new piece of clinical technology was generally well established; however, this case identified that the introduction of a 'replacement' or 'upgraded' model of the same equipment/device was not as thoroughly reviewed, prior to being used. In particular, the differences between the two models in terms of the required monitoring and use of safety alarms were not identified.
6. The role of 'third-party' representatives in procedural areas in terms of their training, education, and proficiencies in the use of medical devices was not thoroughly monitored, discussed, or governed. The training experience of such medical device representatives varies significantly, and no centralised 'accreditation', 'scope of practice', or assessment of such individuals was in place.
7. Insurance and professional indemnity issues were raised because of the inconsistency in the 'management' of such representatives and the potential risk to the organisation and to patient care from a governance perspective.
8. The maintenance records of equipment, particularly if equipment is 'loaned' for a particular surgical procedure (i.e. 'brought in for use by the team by an external company' or 'on-loan' and held within the theatres), were incomplete. It was noted that the governance of such equipment varied across facilities and sites of the same health service and was without a clear centrally coordinated process. Contracts for the maintenance of equipment and for the use of loan equipment require careful monitoring and clear responsibilities for ensuring timely replacement, testing, and routine maintenance.
9. Notification of the introduction of a new piece of equipment, including an upgraded model, was inconsistent and lacked coordination.

This case highlights the importance of a comprehensive, coordinated and, where necessary, centralised investigation of a clinical incident. It highlights the important role played by those involved in clinical equipment procurement, supply, and commissioning, and the necessity to have clear governance accountabilities and responsibilities for the introduction of medical equipment. The training, familiarisation, and experience of clinicians in undertaking procedures and their use of medical equipment is essential to be assessed. It is also critical to ensure that this performance is monitored, and outcomes evaluated and recorded. Reliance on 'previous' experience in such cases can be misleading and can provide a false sense of security.

The need to have ongoing dialogue with regulatory bodies, agencies, manufacturers, and other clinicians is also highlighted. It is particularly important during an investigation of an incident to provide timely and accurate information to patients and their families.

4.3 Case Study 3: Failure to Escalate Deteriorating Patient

A 48-year-old male presented to the emergency department of a large private hospital in the late afternoon on a public holiday with a significant injury sustained as a result of a motorbike accident. Following resuscitation in the emergency room, the patient was transferred to the operating room to undergo surgery to repair the injuries, which were primarily related to fractures of the long bones. The 'on-call' team included a senior surgeon well-known at the hospital who performs many operations, mainly elective procedures. The anaesthetist on call was relatively junior and had not worked with the surgeon previously, and whilst they had previously worked at the same hospital, they were not well known to each other. The anaesthetist was credentialed to be part of the on-call roster and periodically also worked at other hospitals.

During the operation, the patient suffered extreme blood loss, subsequently arrested, and he unfortunately died in the Intensive Care Unit within 24 hours of presenting.

At the time of death, the clinical governance responsibilities for mortality review were unclear, and the complexities of overall governance in a private hospital added to the confusion. Most importantly, this lack of clarity with regards to governance responsibilities pitted clinicians against each other and against the hospital.

The role of the clinical speciality unit and its director was also unclear. The relevant clinical mortality and morbidity meeting did not have the authority or accountability to independently review cases, or to question clinicians about their clinical decisions, and therefore could not comment on the sequence of events that led to the inability to adequately resuscitate the patient and possibly prevent the arrest.

Nursing staff had advised that they were concerned regarding the interactions between the medical staff in the operating theatre during the operation. When questioned, they said there was virtually no communication between the doctors at the time. Despite the operation lasting more than 5 hours, the complexity and deterioration of the clinical situation, the patient's clinical instability and increasing clinical risk appeared to not have been recognised or escalated.

4.3.1 Standard Case Management

This case highlights the importance of an investigation having clear lines of responsibilities and accountabilities that enable thorough analysis and review of the circumstances of an incident. At a minimum, the requirements should include:

1. A coordinated case investigation led by a trained professional working within the clinical governance system of the hospital.
2. The need for an initial 'Immediate Action Meeting' to ensure that the sequence of events/process of investigation is clear from the outset.
3. The requirement to obtain detailed clinical reports from all those who had been involved, to enable a 'sequence of events' to be determined, and for the investigation to progress appropriately.
4. Involvement of the patient, or in the case of death, their family, from the commencement of the investigation and a commitment of ongoing open disclosure with them.
5. The importance of external independent clinical review and expert opinions to enable the investigation team to identify causative issues, target improvements, and focus attention on identifying meaningful solutions.

4.3.2 Patient-centric Incident Case Management

Power dynamics between clinicians can pose a major clinical risk and lead to poor channels of communication, subsequent confusion, and failure to escalate concerns.

Such power dynamics may be 'overt' and involve aggressive, arrogance, and/or overbearing demeanours. In such circumstances , the 'tone' set by that individual can intimidate other clinicians, resulting in a failure to speak up for patient safety, communicate their concerns, and facilitate open disclosure. Such individuals are often well-known and, if tolerated within the hospital system, can cause significant harm, including psychological harm, to those they work with.

However, not all power dynamics have to be overt. Disruptive behaviour in medicine can be displayed in more subtle manners.

There is an unwritten expectation, but present nonetheless, that individual clinicians are 'capable' and 'can manage' all situations. Non-verbal cues between clinicians, particularly at difficult times, can have a significant impact on the confidence and response of junior clinicians who witness these. The use of what may be considered 'non-aggressive phrases', such as 'Are you in control? What's going on?' can have a significant intimidatory psychological impact.

Whilst the tone set between clinicians is everyone's responsibility, it rests more substantively on the most senior clinician present in a situation. Under the Patient-Centric Incident management framework the case was investigated and the following was identified:

In this case, the power dynamic between the anaesthetist and the surgeon was complicated by several significant issues.

The pressure of after-hours on-call/emergency situations can add a high level of complexity to a clinical situation. Therefore, there is a need for a very clear pre-procedure surgical/anaesthetic plan to be developed and discussed, that enables all practitioners to be 'on the same page'. This ensures that in the event of clinical deterioration or unanticipated clinical event, which invariably occurs, that open lines of communication exist, and that each person present feel comfortable enough to voice any concerns and be heard. Establishing such an expectation and 'tone' is essential, it cannot just be assumed to exist by default. Teams that work together regularly often find a 'rhythm' to how procedures are undertaken; however, as seen in this case, it is important not to assume that everyone will feel able to escalate concerns and speak freely. Setting this tone is vital, must be explicit and repeated prior to commencing a case/list. In the circumstances of the case described here, the need for explicit setting of the tone is even more important as the surgical team was not as familiar with each other. Similar to the airline industry, the importance of establishing an expectation and tone where anyone can raise concerns at any time, including stopping what is taking place if necesarry, is very important.

When team members are unfamiliar with each other, or may not have worked with each other frequently, or indeed ever, again like the airline industry, where this situation is not uncommon, it is essential that 'routine processes' are in place to mitigate risks, e.g., surgical safety checklists, and that these are based on open, ongoing communication between individuals.

In this case, a number of points of failure were able to be quickly identified through the IAM:

1. Lack of familiarity between clinicians and a lack of open discussion and channels of communication meant that as clinical deterioration and instability were occurring, updates was not shared, concerns were not raised, and the opportunities for amending the clinical plan were not considered.
2. Assumptions on clinical experience and expertise were made and therefore not discussed, i.e. level of experience in the management of trauma cases and in rapidly changing clinical scenarios which, although can occur in any situation, are predictably more likely in emergency situations unless a clinician is regularly practising in this area. In such a situation, this can pose a significant clinical challenge. Therefore, if clinicians find themselves in such situations, it is essential that the experience and expertise of each are clarified, and a discussion of the possible complex clinical complications that may arise takes place. In addition, a plan for early communication of changes in clinical circumstances should be made and, as necessary, triggers for additional support, e.g. massive transfusion activation, assistance from ICU, etc., are considered ahead of time. The senior clinician must ensure that everyone present is comfortable to raise concerns. The lack of ongoing open discussions, as seen in this case, can lead to significant risk.
3. This case also highlights that, although a clinician may be senior and highly experienced, their scope of practice, e.g. familiarity with trauma cases, needs to be regularly assessed, and that appointment to on-call rosters where trauma cases may be likely, is a specific undertaking after ensuring that skills in this area of clinical practice are recent and can be maintained. There is significant pressure and an expectation on senior clinicians to be able to 'handle' all clinical situa-

tions. In this case, the need to be able to recognise that the clinical situation is not progressing as anticipated, and that a modification to the plan was necessary, required significant reflection, judgement, and an element of humility, all of which unfortunately were absent in this case.

Once the clinician has set the tone of open communication, they are then required to 'listen' and 'hear' the concerns of their colleagues, reassess the situation, seek comments and opinions from them, and call for assistance if required. In some cases, this may include 'abandoning' the clinical plan in place due to the changing clinical situation, and includes recognition that their plan may have 'failed'. Persisting with the plan in such cases may lead to poor outcomes.

Senior clinicians need to be aware of their own changing clinical experience and practice, and request consequent adjustments to their scope of practice. Whilst the organisation needs to have systems in place to ensure that individuals maintain recency in their scopes of practice, e.g. in order to participate in after-hours roster cover, individual clinicians also need to assess their own clinical practice and determine when to make necessary changes based on their recency of practice.

Speaking up were there is safety concerns is a fundamental tenet of clinical governance. In this case, whilst a number of clinicians were aware of the rapidly changing clinical scenario and were concerned that insufficient action was taking place, there was a lack of advocacy for the patient and a lack of confidence to raise their concerns. In addition to the 'tone' mentioned above, senior clinicians 'on the floor' aware of the deteriorating clinical scenario, specifically did not act directly or escalate their concerns. The opportunity to advocate for the patient, provide additional resources, and call for assistance was therefore lost.

As clinical governance processes were not well-developed, the lack of a coordinated review following the incident resulted in a considerable impact on all clinicians. A lack of confidence in the clinical governance system and lack of transparency in the process meant that the clinicians did not access the supports that were available to them, resulting in ongoing self-doubt and feelings of guilt. This led to reinforcement of the notion that 'nothing will be done', in future similar scenarios.

To counter the negative consequences of the investigation that had occurred, a 'Patient-centric Incident management' approach was undertaken some six months after the event. This recognised the long-term impact on culture, morale, and confidence of staff of an inadequately managed investigation, and that although delayed, it was essential to 'start afresh' and complete a thorough, open investigative process.

Firstly, establishing a clear 'just culture' approach to the investigation, undertaken from a Patient-Centric perspective, and focusing on improving clinical care, and implementing improvement practices, is essential. Therefore, the following was undertaken:

- Reinterviewing clinicians concerned, in addition to the clinical details and taking the opportunity to discuss concerns about the 'tone', communication, operating plan, and the response to changing clinical scenarios.

- Discussing individual scope of practice, particularly recency of practice and adequacy of performing on-call trauma work.
- Clarifying the role of clinical audit, particularly, morbidity and mortality meetings, clinician reviews, and clinical discussions, ensuring transparency in such processes.
- Obtaining independent expert opinions from a surgeon and anaesthetist who discussed the case with the clinicians involved to gain clarity and insight into opportunities for improvement.
- Discussing escalation and notification of clinical deteriorations to ensure additional resources are activated, and to provide what is needed directly to where care is provided.
- Establishing clear senior authority within the hospital at all hours to intervene in such clinical scenarios, to overcome any resistance to help and focus on the patient.
- Re-engaging the family and advising on changes to the investigation process, inviting their participation and committing to ongoing open disclosure and regular updates.
- Engaging with regulatory bodies involved and advising on the renewed investigation and a commitment to implementing recommendations and other actions.
- Using the case as an example of reframing clinical governance in the organisation with a focus on patient-centric clinical incident investigation, contemporary open disclosure, patient/family involvement, transparency, and a focus on just culture and commitment to improvement.

There is a significant degree of clinician stress and anxiety when a case is revisited/reinvestigated, and there may be a tendency to become defensive, adversarial, and suspicious. Therefore, this requires significant planning, openness, and clarity of purpose with a focus on a 'just culture' and with emphasis on the importance of the opportunity for improvement to enable cooperation between all parties and to create a sense of shared purpose.

Medical indemnity insurers need to be engaged, so that they can support their practitioners and at the same time encourage their open and honest contribution and involvement in the process.

A commitment to improve the process of investigation and incident management on the part of those responsible for clinical governance, is particularly essential.

4.4 Case Study 4: Clinical Service Line Failure

A hospital group is advised by the jurisdictional regulatory safety body that it is an outlier in terms of mortality outcomes in complex surgical cases. The agency meets with the organisation and provides benchmark data that shows the variance in mortality compared with similar organisations. The agency advises it is considering enforcing a closure of the hospital Group's services in this speciality, and that this decision will depend upon the action the hospital group will take and the degree of sense of urgency demonstrated in terms of the Group's reponse. In view of the well-publicised clinical governance failures in the past across the jurisdiction, the agency explains the importance of a sense of urgency and concerns for safety as being paramount. Whilst the loss of the service would have significant reputational and financial repercussions, the issue of safety and the data presented is a clear and present clinical and reputational risk.

4.4.1 Standard Case Management

On receiving the data, the following actions were commenced:

1. Review of data provided against the data held by the hospital. This included:
   - Activity by doctor, site, procedure, volume, length of stay, re-admissions, and transfers.
   - Clinical outcomes such as hospital-acquired complications (infections, unplanned ICU admissions, etc.).
   - Mortality in hospital.
2. Review of practitioner credentialing, and scope of practice against procedures undertaken.
3. Comparison with relevant national/state outcome registry data.
4. Internal outcomes benchmarked by individual, and across various campuses of the group.
5. Use of clinical pathways, e.g. antibiotic prophylaxis, DVT prevention, and similar
6. Review of clinical guidelines regarding recommendations of treatment options and 'gold standard care'.

4.4.2 Patient-Centric Incident Case Management

In addition to the above process, the senior executive responsible for clinical governance called for an IAM, and directed an immediate establishment of clinical criteria for approval of a the type of cases in question before proceeding to surgery. This included a requirement for obtaining a formal second opinion regarding appropriateness of surgery, a formal peri-op medical consultation, ICU consultation, and consults from any other relevant clinical speciality as indicated. A formal approval process for ensuring this was then established, followed by the requirement for a comprehensive post-operative case report and clinical outcome report to be submitted.

Additional clinical governance improvements were implemented:

1. Establishment of a Multidisciplinary Meeting (MDM) to ensure that best practice decision-making is in place for each case, with a formal requirement for case presentations and reaching of consensus opinion, with subsequent communication of the decision to all clinicians involved as well as the patient.

2. Establishment of an ongoing compliance audit, and communication and follow up with any clinicians not complying with these requirements.
3. Communication of the change in process requiring approval and MDM involvement, to key stakeholders within the organisation, e.g. bookings, theatre teams, and clinical safety and quality teams was undertaken.
4. Communication with medical practitioners clearly outlining the concerns raised by the agency, inviting clinicians input, cooperation, collaboration, insights, and responding to concerns while incorporating their ideas and suggestions.
5. Conducting practitioner meetings with those whose activity and recency of practice indicate that changes to their scope of practice should be considered.
6. Reviewing each mortality case to identify individual case-specific issues and any broad system-wide issues being made a formal requirement.
7. Identifying if alternative treatment options should have been considered was incorporated in this process. Communication with clinicians and involving them in this process was seen as critical.

Further, reviewing all support clinical programs that are in place to provide complex surgical care, and benchmarking against similar programs was considered essential. This included radiology, particularly the availability of after-hours interventional radiology, ICU, emergency department, pathology, and pharmacy. The role of peri-operative physicians, anaesthetists, and subspeciality physicians, e.g. respiratory and cardiology, who are essential to ensure that the patient's fitness for surgery was maximised. This was to ensure that postoperative complications could be anticipated and mitigation strategies be put in place. A review of nursing expertise in surgical, recovery, and post-surgical ward-based care, especially the early identification of critical post-operative complications and the escalation of these concerns and issues was also completed. Other key components that were assessed included:

- The availability of specialist expertise/cover, over a 24/7 period that can be contacted and escalated to in relation to emerging concerns, and the identification of individuals who were credentialed to provide such care if they were not the primary surgeon.
- The pre-arranging of post-surgical care, including ICU, routine diagnostics, and use of established clinical pathways.
- The rapid response to emergency complications and concerns including any critical diagnostic testing.
- Assurance that the clinical plan is known and understood by all.

From a Patient-Centric Incident management it was apparent that the involvement of the patient and their family in the planning process, including at the MDM, and peri-operative reviews, and the capacity for the patient and family to escalate any concerns they may have at any time in their care journey was insufficient and needed to be addressed.

Case review at clinical audit/mortality and morbidity meetings require an inter-speciality and multidisciplinary approach, including the other key specialities as outlined above, with agreed clinical outcomes that are to be measured and benchmarked.

Ensuring that the appropriate clinical equipment, e.g. monitoring, navigational, and radiological, particularly in the theatre complex, is in place to maximise clinical outcomes is essential. There is a balance between what is needed by the clinicians to provide best care versus the pressure for investing in the newest technology. This is despite the evidence for the need and benefit of such equipment not always being available at times, and therefore healthcare leaders needing to consider completing demands.

Establishing regular morbidity and mortality meetings, and engaging practitioners in the process for immediate review of significant complications and incorporation of these as part of the incident management system, was a particularly focal aspect.

4.5 Case Study 5: Failure of Reporting

A 57-year-old male patient was admitted to hospital for chemotherapy treatment the night before, as he was from a regional area and could not attend on the same day of the procedure. In the morning prior to treatment commencing, the patient was seen by the oncologist and the treating team. He was generally well but described a short period of chest pain and dyspnoea.

The patient was noted to have a slightly raised temperature which was determined to be due to a respiratory infection, for which antibiotics were commenced. A chest X-ray and ECG were arranged, and performed within an hour. The patient's symptoms, particularly the chest discomfort, then resolved.

Subsequently, the patient was seen by a therapist approximately 2 hours later. He reported feeling nauseated and dizzy, the therapist ceased the treatment and advised the treating team.

Shortly after, the patient stated he felt better as he was resting. However, within the next hour, the patient's condition suddenly deteriorated, and he suffered a cardiac arrest and died.

The clinical team explained to the family that although this was an unexpected death, as he had been admitted for elective chemotherapy, the death was likely due to an underlying cardiac condition resulting in a heart attack.

Whilst tragic, there was deemed to be no evidence of any failure in care; the autopsy confirmed a heart attack, and this information was passed on to the family and treating team. The mortality review of the case determined that the clinical scenario was unpredictable and it was fortuitous that he was in the hospital at the time when he would otherwise have been at home and would have suffered the heart attack there.

The mortality review noted that the patient's symptoms at the time of the clinical assessment were consistent with the diagnosis of chest infection and that appropriate investigations and management had taken place. The review determined that apart from a few minor issues, the investigation could be closed.

A junior medical director who had been recently assigned to the hospital, reviewed the investigation as a matter of routine. She noted that an ECG had been performed and that it appeared to indicate evidence of a myocardial infarction (MI). There was no evidence that the ECG had been reviewed by the clinical team or that the MI had been identified prior to the patient's death.

Following the identification of these issues, she approached the initial review team and advised that the case should be reopened, and a formal notification of a potentially avoidable death be made to the coroner. There was initial resistance to this from the review team as:

1. It was known and accepted that the patient already had a malignancy with a potential poor diagnosis.
2. The hospital did not have its own angioplasty service, and that as the patient died shortly after symptoms were reported, there would not have been any change in the clinical management, and even had the ECG been reviewed, it would therefore not have changed his outcome.

4.5.1 Standard Mortality Review

The original clinical mortality review process that was undertaken confirmed the clinician's position that the clinical scenario was unpredictable, and therefore the death was not preventable. The patient's familywere advised that the death was unexpected and not preventable.

4.5.2 Patient-Centric Incident Management Approach

Despite what appeared to be a straightforward clinical scenario, this case demonstrates the importance of a rigorous mortality review process that is free of 'confirmation bias'. This also highlights the need to be prepared to review a decision at any time when and if new information becomes available.

In this case, the medical director arranged for the ECG to be reviewed by an independent cardiologist who confirmed an acute infarct had been present at the time the ECG was recorded, which was 30 min after the initial oncologist review.

Unfortunately, the ECG had not been reviewed by any of the clinicians involved in the care of the patient during his admission. The ECG was reviewed within an hour by an 'offsite' contracted medical practitioner, who had noted the abnormality, however a result was not provided to the treating team.

The medical director commissioned an IAM which directed that a new incident investigation using Root Cause Analysis (RCA) methodology be undertaken. The patient's family were advised of the new information and actively engaged in the investigation. The IAM also directed that all ECGs be reviewed immediately, and the offsite medical practitioner was mandated to escalate any abnormalities in an ECG to the treating clinicians immediately as part of routine process.

The RCA determined that a number of key changes in the management of chest pain would need to be put in place, including direct access to another hospital's cardiac catheter laboratory. These improvements subsequently were activated in similar clinical scenarios at the hospital with good patient outcomes.

From a clinical governance perspective, however, several improvements to the process of incident review were also required:

1. Avoiding confirmation bias when reviewing cases, and ensuring independence, thoroughness, and transparency of investigations.
2. A strong culture of safety and quality, along with a desire to improve being essential to ensure that all incidents are reviewed based on the merits of the case and that patient's families are involved in the process.
3. The acceptance that such a culture also welcomes an opportunity to conduct subsequent reviews based on the identification of additional information, and that it encourages clinicians, and others, to integrate data and information, until they are satisfied that the correct determination has been made.

As part of the review, it was important to advise the patient's family that new information had been identified and that there had been a missed opportunity to intervene and change the outcome their loved one suffered.

Due to the seriousness of the implications of this information and the expected impact on the family, a senior clinical executive undertook the disclosure of this information in person, and apologised for both the clinical care and the delay in advising the family. The active involvement of the family in the second investigation had a significant positive impact. Engaging them in the subsequent outcome actions and involving them in seeing how developing the changes to the processes at the hospital would prevent recurrence of a similar clinical situation, was received well by the family.

The case also highlighted the importance of personal integrity and professionalism. Following the 'majority decision' without question is often the more 'straightforward' option, whilst challenging decisions of senior staff can be often very confronting and anxiety-producing. Therefore, embedding a proactive culture and supporting team members to speak up, to be heard, to be encouraged, and to expect challenging inquiries as the norm, is essential.

Further Reading

Delivering High Quality Healthcare – Victorian Clinical Governance Framework: Department of Health Victoria (2017).

McSherry R and Pearce P. Clinical Governance: A guide to implementation for healthcare professionals. Third Edition. 2010.

Chambers, Ruth, et al. Clinical effectiveness and clinical governance made easy. 4th edition. 2007.

Brennan, Niamh and Flynn, Maureen A. Differentiating clinical governance, clinical management and clinical practice. Clinical Governance 2013; 18 (2): 114–131

Swage T. Clinical Governance in healthcare practice. Second Edition. 2003.

Gottwald M. Clinical governance: Improving the quality of healthcare for patients and service users. Second Edition. 2021.

Haxby E et al. An introduction to clinical governance and patient safety. 2010.

McConnell C. Case studies in healthcare supervision. Second Edition. 2011.

Clinical Excellence Queensland. Best practice guide to clinical incident management. First Edition. 2014.

Australian Commission on Safety and Quality in Health Care. Incident Management Guide. Sydney: ACSQHC; 2021.

5 Contemporary Open Disclosure

Open disclosure (OD) is the open discussion of adverse events that resulted in harm to a patient whilst receiving care, and it is conducted with the patient, their families, and carers. Key elements of OD should include a genuine apology or expression of regret, and it should include the words 'I am sorry' or 'we are sorry', a factual explanation of what happened, and finally, an opportunity for the patient, their family, and carers to relate their experience of what occurred during the incident.

There should then be a discussion of the potential consequences of the adverse event for the patient, and an explanation of the steps being taken to manage the adverse event and prevent its recurrence.

It is important to acknowledge that OD is not a one-way provision of information. It is a *discussion* between the healthcare representatives, the patient, and their family, and involves an exchange of information, and may take several meetings over a period of time.

Leaders are key in developing a safe and just culture and need to foster a culture where people feel supported and encouraged to identify and report adverse events so that the opportunity for system improvements can be identified, acted on, and shared. It is imperative that leaders create a culture where patients, their families and carers, clinicians, and managers all feel supported.

In *Patient-Centric Incident Management (PCIM)* ©, communication is key. Effective communication with the patient commences at the beginning of an episode of care and continues throughout the duration of care. There is an ethical responsibility for clinicians to maintain honest and open communication with the patient, their families, and carers, especially if care does not go according to plan.

Essential to PCIM is ensuring that feedback is provided to the patient, family, and carers. Recommendations from incident investigations should also be passed on to the family and carers. Preceding this they should be informed about the progress of investigations throughout the process. They should be invited to participate in the investigation, pose questions to the investigating team, raise concerns with regards to any issues that have been identified, and be able to comment on the findings and

© The Author(s), under exclusive license to Springer Nature Singapore Pte Ltd. 2026

L. Prado, S. Chandrasiri, *The Practice of Clinical Governance*,
https://doi.org/10.1007/978-981-19-7896-8_5

recommendations. Finally, they should have a commitment provided to them that the recommendations will be enacted.

As part of PCIM, it is important that practical support for patients, their families, and carers to cope with the effects of harm is provided. This can include reimbursement or covering of out-of-pocket expenses, in particular, including the cost of items the patient might require as a consequence of the harm that occurred.

Open disclosure in PCIM can fail, and there are a number of reasons for this that commonly occur. The first is that there is a delay in the commencement of the Open Disclosure process following the incident, and therefore a delay in the acknowledgement of the harm to the patient. Whilst there is no clear timing in terms of the impact on a patient, the general rule is that Open Disclosure occurs as soon as practically possible. Once the incident has been identified, an acknowledgement of the harm should be made by the most senior person available in the organisation and those treating the patient at that time.

Open disclosure is sometimes seen by clinicians as a 'once-off' event, but this is not the case. If it is undertaken as a once-off event, patients then feel 'deserted'; and this can result in the entire process being found 'wanting' by the patient. If clinicians and leaders do not appear to be listening to the patient, not acknowledging that harm has occurred, and/or not saying sorry, this can lead to the patient and their family feeling that the process is not genuine and sincere, and can disconnect them from it entirely.

It is essential to allow the patient the opportunity to tell their story and to be heard. The process can fall apart when it appears to have been done for the clinician or for the organisation as the key driver, rather than for the patient. If the patient does not receive ongoing, continuous communication, they can feel deserted by the organisation, which can then lead to greater distress and distrust.

5.1 Case Study 1: Escalating Adverse Patient Incident

The Chief Medical Officer (CMO) is contacted on a Sunday morning by the Hospital Coordinator (HC). The HC advises that one of the porters of the hospital wishes to speak to the CMO about an urgent matter.

The porter comes to the phone and advises that a few hours earlier, when transferring a patient from the ICU to the radiology department for an MRI, he had removed his metal earrings and had placed them for safe keeping in a barrel of a 5 mL syringe.

Whilst he is not certain, he feels it is possible that the same syringe had been used to draw up a saline flush and had been used to flush the patient's central lines. He wanted to advise the CMO, that in addition to this issue, that he is Hepatitis C positive and HIV positive, and that this was not known by the organisation.

On receiving this information, the CMO contacts the ICU team on the phone, advises them of the clinical scenario as described by the porter, maintaining confidentiality of the individual's identity, and advises the initial actions that would need to take place. The CMO advises she will be present in the unit within 45 min. Once on-site, she checks and confirms the status of the patient as being 'stable' and that there had not been any immediate consequences from the potential contamination.

On arrival, the CMO meets with the patient and their family. She advises them of the circumstances as described, apologises to them, and ensures through the clinicians that the appropriate clinical care, including infectious diseases review and follow-up pathology testing, and other preventative measures, are put in place. Subsequently, the patient remains stable and over a period of months does not suffer any clinical consequences from the incident.

However, for approximately 3 months, the patient and their family are extremely anxious with regards to the risk that they had been exposed to and the potential consequences of transmission of infection.

Whilst the infectious diseases specialist had advised that the risks were very low, they could not be excluded, and although reassured, the patient remains very concerned. The CMO maintains regular contact with the patient, ensures that all costs for provision of testing and other elements of care are covered, and that all out-of-pocket costs for the previous care episode are reimbursed. In addition, the patient's costs for transport and accommodation to undertake the subsequent reviews with specialists are also covered by the hospital.

Formal apologies are provided to the patient at the time and subsequently throughout the process, and the patient and their family are engaged as part of the clinical review investigation.

The family is advised of the outcome of the review and given an opportunity to review the outcomes, recommendations, and actions. Following the implementation of these recommendations, they are advised of the monitoring process that is put in place to ensure that similar events would not happen again.

The patient and family make comments to the CMO that they recognised that had there not been a culture of escalating to the CMO of a significant clinical risk by the staff members, no one would have been the wiser in this situation. It was acknowledged that an organisational culture where a staff member feels capable of contacting the CMO directly at a critical time in the patient's care indicates that there is a strong culture of patient safety.

Although the incident itself was preventable, the fact that the information had been provided swiftly and escalated early and then presented to the patient and their family and acted upon, is seen favourably by the patient and their family.

There is much investigation, research and analysis that overwhelmingly shows that the factual and transparent communication of adverse events and the subsequent investigation's findings and improvements with an appropriate apology or expression of regret has a positive impact on patients, protects the clinician's and the organisations' reputation and reduces medico-legal risk. Despite this, there remains significant reluctance to fully adopt genuine open disclosure as part of routine clinical care. Whilst most patients experience good outcomes, adverse events do occur in clinical practice, and the impact of such incidents goes beyond the direct clinical outcomes. These can include anxiety, loss of trust and faith in healthcare providers, unexpected financial burden and potential long-term impacts on health and other social aspects including employment, for patients, their families and friends.

As stated above, Open disclosure (OD) is the process of communicating with patients and their families about adverse events that is now considered a fundamental component of delivering ethical, high-quality, and safe healthcare. Effective OD is also critical for rebuilding patient trust and is key to creating a culture of improvement and learning within healthcare organisations. Teaching OD to clinicians is a complex matter, as many can feel that their clinical practice is being questioned when required to undertake such training. Many also can feel that the OD is already incorporated within their clinical practice as 'how they do things now', and that they do not need to be 'told how to speak to (their) patients'.

Whilst OD needs to be conducted in an authentic manner and should avoid a 'scripted' approach to the communicating the details of the incident, it is advisable that clinicians are taught some structure in undertaking the OD discussion to ensure that the critical elements are not inadvertently missed. In a similar vein, although clinicians may feel that they are already excellent communicators, training in how to provide information in an honest and ethical manner that responds to the patient's emotional state and that helps the clinician adapt to potential challenging interactions, is very important. Critical components of the OD process include:

- Prompt acknowledgment: Initiating contact with the patient and/or family as soon as possible after an adverse event.
- Factual explanation: Providing a clear and honest explanation of what happened, using language that is easily understood.
- Expression of regret: Offering a sincere apology and acknowledging the impact of the event on the individual.
- Opportunity for questions and dialogue: Creating a safe space for the patient and/or family to ask questions and express their concerns.
- Commitment to improvement: Outlining the steps taken or planned to prevent similar incidents from occurring in the future.

Despite this, challenges to the conducting of high-quality OD continue to be observerd. These include:

1. Clinicians not understanding that their view of 'known complications' and the patients' expectations of clinical outcomes may not always align, and may represent different perspectives as to what is accepted as 'standard of care'.
2. The emotional impact on the clinician who is conducting OD can often be unrecognised or undervalued and therefore considerable harm can occur to the clinicians involved in the case, including loss of confidence and ability to work.
3. Clinician's concerns regarding medico-legal implications and requirements for reporting to regulatory bodies and other agencies, such as the coroner.
4. Lack of support from healthcare leaders, including focusing their concerns on organisational reputation and insurance impact, may result in clinicians being reluctant to undertake OD within such unsupportive organisational cultures.

Therefore, in acknowledging that such issues remain and recognising these challenges, embedding contemporary open disclosure within a healthcare organisation can be greatly assisted by the following strategies:

1. Comprehensive training programs for healthcare providers on communication skills, empathic listening, and conflict resolution. Such training should include understanding emotional responses, both in the patient and in the clinician, as well as understanding how to manage an OD meeting if the tone or interactions begin to deteriorate as a result.
2. Involving and having the support of the healthcare leadership, including the board and executive, with understanding the importance of OD is critical. Similarly, involving and having the support of other clinicians, quality and risk managers, legal counsel, and patient advocates, is instrumental in to embedding a culture of authentic OD in the organisation.
3. Collecting and analysing outcome data on open disclosure meetings, including receiving patient, family and clinician feedback, is important, and can identify key areas for improvement or modification, and inform on-going practice.
4. Ensuring that when planning for the OD meeting, the clinicians are aware of the patient's cultural, spiritual, and personal values and preferences.
5. It is critical that OD is incorporated into the broader patient safety and quality improvement process, and that lessons learned from adverse events make meaningful improvements to to clinical care.
6. Leaders should ensure that their support is made available and accessible to both clinicians and patients and their families, as part of the OD process, including on an ongoing basis after the meeting, as required. Consideration of a peer support network that is equipped to provide this support may also be important.
7. Whilst some elements of OD training can be undertaken via didactic sessions and on-line learning, the best method of OD training is a commitment to simulation and 'role-play' scenarios that can provide a practical and realistic experience of what the actual impact of OD can be. This allows clinicians to practise their communication skills in a safe environment and to continue to improve them in response to feedback received.

5.2 Case Study 2: Communication Failure

Following a significant unexpected surgical complication from a retained surgical gauze in a 28-year-old woman who underwent an elective bowel procedure, the safety and quality manager met with the surgeon to plan the OD meeting to be undertaken. This discussion was intended to include planning for providing an apology to the patient, and advising them of the outcomes of the Root Cause Analysis (RCA) investigation that was undertaken, including the improvements that were planned to be made.

The surgeon, who was the previous department director and one of the hospital's most senior clinicians, sent a late cancellation to this OD planning meeting, but advised he would still attend the actual OD meeting with the patient. He stated that he was comfortable to do so as he was fully briefed on the investigation and that he had an excellent relationship with the patient. He also advised that he was not at all concerned about how the meeting would transpire. Unfortunately, the surgeon was delayed getting to the actual OD meeting due to a theatre list that had run late, and the meeting had to commence without him. The safety and quality manager was explaining the OD process and outlining the investigation undertaken and the findings at the time when the surgeon arrived at the meeting. On entering the room, the surgeon promptly sat down on the vacant chair, and without any form of introduction, proclaimed this was the most distressing and serious issue that had happened to him in his 30 years of practice. The patient's father then in response, stated: "so you have had a dirty piece of gauze left behind in your abdomen too have you? You have suffered pain and been unable to work and lost income and can't look after your children too? Well you must have, if you're saying you have suffered like my daughter". This case highlights that regardless of clinical expertise and knowledge, OD remains a complex and emotional process, and to be effective and meaningful requires a great deal of training and preparation.

Further Reading

Safer Care Victoria. Victorian Duty of Candour Framework: an implementation guide. 2022.

Australian Commission on Safety and Quality in HealthCare. Australian Open Disclosure Framework, 2013.

Harrison R, Walton M, Smith-Merry J, Manias E, Iedema R. Open disclosure of adverse events: exploring the implications of service and policy structures on practice. Risk Manag Health Policy. 2019 Jan 23;12:5–12.

Wojcieszak D et al. Sorry works! Disclosure, apology and relationships to prevent medical malpractice claims. 2007.

Bruckner, Hilda J, and Woods, Michael S. Healing Words: The Power of Apology in Medicine. United States, Doctors in Touch, 2004.

Iedema R et al.; Communicating Quality and safety in healthcare. 2015

Clinical Governance in Medical Workforce Management

6

Clinical governance within medical workforce management is paramount for ensuring patient safety and quality of care. Effective systems should incorporate clear lines of accountability, robust performance monitoring, and regular professional development opportunities. This involves not only credentialing and appraisal processes but also the implementation of policies that support ethical practice and continuous improvement. Further, proactive risk management strategies and transparent reporting mechanisms are crucial for identifying and addressing potential issues before they impact patient outcomes, fostering a culture of learning and accountability within the medical team.

6.1 Credentialing and Defining Scope of Practice

A system for the credentialing of all health care professionals is required across most countries and jurisdictions and are operational at varying levels of maturity. In this chapter, the Australian context is used as an example, as is the process for the appointment of medical practitioners. The process detailed in this chapter is applicable across all jurisdictions and professional groups. In Australia, hospitals must be accredited by an independent accreditation agency such as the *Australian Council on HealthCare Standards (ACHS)*, in order to operate and receive public funding (public health services). Private health services must also be accredited in order to be licensed and to be able to enter into health purchasing and funding agreements with private health insurers.

Hospital accreditation is a process that assesses a hospital's performance against a set of standards and benchmarks, and is intended to promote continuous improvement in the quality of care provided by the hospital. Periodic accreditation requirements against the *National Safety and Quality Health Services (NSQHS) Standards* are designed to ensure that hospitals provide high-quality care to patients and protect their health and wellbeing.

© The Author(s), under exclusive license to Springer Nature Singapore Pte Ltd. 2026

L. Prado, S. Chandrasiri, *The Practice of Clinical Governance*,
https://doi.org/10.1007/978-981-19-7896-8_6

Standard 1 of NSQHS: Clinical Governance requires health services to implement a clinical governance framework that ensures a system of appropriate governance, leadership, and culture at all levels, which ensures patient safety and quality systems are in place to allow a safe environment for the delivery of care. It further specifies that the clinical workforce has the right qualifications, skills and appropriate supervision where required, to provide safe care, through a process to credential and define the scope of practice for clinicians, that is in alignment with the clinical service capacity of the organisation and against the health services' clinical services plan.

Credentialing and defining the scope of practice are important components of the relationship between hospitals and the doctors who provide care to patients in those facilities. The provision of safe and clinically appropriate healthcare by health practitioners is an expectation of the public for all patients treated in public or private health services. Health service organisations are required to appoint health practitioners who are suitably experienced, trained, and qualified to practise in a competent and ethical manner in accordance with service needs and organisational capabilities (*Australian Commission on Safety and Quality in Health Care* 2015).

Credentialing refers to the formal process used to verify the qualifications, training, experience, competency, professional standing, and other relevant professional attributes of a medical practitioner for the purpose of verifying and evaluating their competence, performance, and professional suitability to provide safe, high-quality healthcare services.

Defining the scope of practice follows on from credentialing and involves delineating the extent of a medical practitioner's clinical practice within the health service, based on their credentials, competence, performance, and professional suitability, as well as the needs and capabilities of the health service to support the requested scope of clinical practice.

Appointment refers to the formal offer and acceptance of a role (in either a staff specialist capacity or an independent contractor capacity) within the health service for a defined period of time in a full or partial capacity. Usually, initial appointments range from 1 to 3 years.

6.2 Developing a Framework for a Credentialing System

Developing a credentialing framework involves creating a structured set of processes, standards, and criteria for evaluating and verifying the qualifications, training, and experience of healthcare professionals. Medical leaders are encouraged to consider the following aspects when setting up their credentialing system and processes:

1. Determine the scope and criteria of the credentialing system: Identify which healthcare professionals will be subject to credentialing and scope of practice processes. For example, junior doctors, who are under the direct supervision of independently practising specialists, may not need detailed definitions of scopes of practice.

2. For Private Health Services: Identify the applicability of credentialing requirements to the various facility arrangements that may exist within private health services. For example:

    (a) Medical practitioners who practise at a facility that is owned, leased, subleased, or licensed on a sessional basis by the private health service provider.
    (b) Medical practitioners who practise on behalf of an independent service provider, such as radiology or pathology clinics providing services to the private health service.

3. Establish a credentialing committee (or equivalent) and/or process that incorporates the right skill set of specialist practitioners with the expertise and experience to assess the various specific aspects required in reviewing credentialing applications. This may involve the establishment of a multi-step process for the various aspects needing review. The aspects that need to be considered include:

    (a) Alignment to facility-based clinical capability.
    (b) Alignment to facility operational and financial capability, e.g. theatre list availability and future plans for business growth, transfer of business to the health service, etc.
    (c) Assessment of formal qualifications, registration(s) with professional bodies, education, and other formal training.
    (d) Assessment of skill, activity levels, experience levels, and recency of practice. This may include logbooks, reference reports, proctor reports, and relevant certifications.
    (e) Assessment of professional suitability and cultural fit with the organisation/facility.
    (f) Compliance with national/state regulations, e.g. working with children checks, medical indemnity insurance, mandatory training requirements, proof of identity, and police checks.
    (g) Requirements for assessing suitability for reappointment, at the expiration of the appointment period, and variations/changes to initially defined scopes of practice.
    (h) Oversight of medical practitioners' clinical practice to ensure compliance with the approved credentials and defined scopes of practice.
    (i) Processes for reviewing a medical practitioner appointment and/or variation to an approved scope of practice should there be any impairment, clinical competence, and/or professional unsuitability during their appointment period.
    (j) A process for appeals to the decision-making pertaining to medical practitioners' credentialing, appointment, performance management, and changes to approved scopes of practice.
    (k) For private health services: Maintaining an appropriate balance between the financial and profit drivers related to clinical activity, resulting from the credentialing and appointment of medical practitioners, and ensuring patient safety remains the cornerstone of credentialing practices.

(l) For private health services: Preventing anti-competitive and/or cartel-behaviour in the appointing of medical practitioners to and within private health services. Ensuring adherence to any advertising guidelines for how appointed medical practitioners promote their services are other aspects that need careful oversight as part of credentialing systems and processes.

4. Establishing a system for facilitating the appointment process is essential. Beginning with how an applicant may express an interest in becoming credentialed at the facility, through to managing and processing the administrative aspects involved, such as collation of documents submitted, maintaining privacy and confidentiality, and an information exchange/communication process between the key stakeholders involved at each step. This should include the process by which healthcare professionals will be notified of their eligibility status, and how their credentials will be maintained. This often involves the utilisation of electronic credentialing software/databases.
5. Ensuring that there is clear governance for ongoing monitoring of the appointment system and process. This includes the development of terms of references for any committees established, delegation matrixes for those involved in approving/endorsing decisions made, and position descriptions for ensuring clear roles and responsibilities.
6. Establishing a review and appeals process. It is important to establish a review and appeals process for medical practitioners who are not approved for appointment or who have their appointment modified or revoked.

6.3 Private Health Services: Credentialing and Defining Scope of Practice

Credentialing committees, whether they function as the overarching decision-maker or is one step of a multi-step credentialing process, are convened in an advisory role within most private health services. Very often, as the medical practitioners of private health services are not employed, this means that credentialing committees may be comprised of individuals who are providing this work in a voluntary capacity. Hence, it is the role of the medical leaders within the private health service who oversee the credentialing system to ensure the committee remains engaged, appropriately skilled, supported and committed to their role.

Credentialing committees must comprise medical practitioners from a range of specialities and must have the option to co-opt additional expertise/advice at any time should it be deemed necessary. This should include community and 'non-medical' committee members where possible.

Medical leaders must ensure that those who are involved in credentialing decision-making, whether as part of a committee or otherwise, remain demonstrably independent with no actual and/or perceived conflicts of interest, propriety interests, and/or any form of commercially conflicting interests with the parties who will be impacted by their advice-provision and/or decision-making.

At the start of each meeting, any such conflicts must be actively sought out, and if any are identified and/or declared, the relevant person(s) will need to be excused from the rest of the meeting or area of decision-making.

There needs to be a clearly outlined Terms of Reference, articulating of the committee functions, and any additional education and training that is to be provided to committee members, to satisfactorily carry out their roles.

Decision-making by the credentialing committee must align with, and ensure natural justice and procedural fairness is applied, be consistent, and any decision-making be based on a merit-basis. Whilst credentialing committees comprised of private medical practitioners may deliberate on the clinical and professional suitability of an applicant, their involvement in aligning credentialing decisions with an organisation's operational, business, reputational, and commercial aspects should be actively discouraged. This is to safeguard against the introduction of potential levels of bias and/or commercial and other conflicts of interest.

Finally, there should be a process established for the formal evaluation and review of committee performance, either via internal and/or external auditing activities.

A private health service's system or process for credentialing and defining the scope of practice requires a realisation that it is an organisational governance responsibility and an important tool with which it can engage its medical workforce. It is also a means by which the relationships that exist between the health service and regulatory bodies, professional registration bodies, speciality colleges, and medical associations can be strengthened and effectively maintained.

Medical leaders of private health organisations must ensure adequate systems and processes exist for:

- Medical practitioner recruitment, which involves matching skills, experience, and qualifications to the role and responsibilities of each position.
- Medical practitioner credentialing and defining their scope of clinical practice.
- Reviewing credentialing and scope of clinical practices as part of reappointment processes.
- Ensuring all established commitments are practised in accordance with the health service's by-laws, policies, and protocols, and codes of conduct. Ensuring that there are adequate processes for allowing sensitive disclosures of adverse findings or other similar matters in relation to the applicant.
- Managing requests for and/or requirements for any changes/variations to existing scopes of clinical practice.
- Performance reviews, peer reviews (or equivalent review processes), and ongoing performance development of all credentialed medical practitioners.
- Orientation and onboarding processes, access to professional support, education, and training, and where appropriate, mentoring and supervision arrangements have been considered and put in place.

A key role of private health service leaders is to determine their service's capacity and capability, by describing the range and scope of clinical services each facility or sites is equipped for and is capable of providing.

This should be reflective of the different levels of patient need and complexity of care that can be provided at each facility. This is crucial in implementing an appropriate framework across which the medical practitioners' skills, knowledge, and qualifications can be matched to and aligned to the specific scope of practice they have been approved to perform at a particular hospital site.

When mapping the framework for determining the type and complexity of services that are being provided at a particular site, health service leaders should have a good understanding of the clinical services plan, the regulatory and licensing requirements, health insurance and funding arrangements, access to technology, equipment, imaging, and laboratory services, existing staffing qualifications and skill mix.

6.4 Relationship Between a Private Hospital and Its Appointed Medical Practitioners

The relationship between a private hospital and appointed doctors can take many forms. The most common arrangement is through a medical practitioner credentialing process and the health service bylaws, however, named. In this process, the hospital evaluates and verifies the qualifications, training, and experience of doctors who wish to practice at the hospital.

The hospital may require doctors to provide proof of medical education, training, certification, licensure, and malpractice/indemnity insurance. Once the credentialing process is complete, the medical practitioner is typically granted *privileges* to practice, i.e. a formal appointment with a defined scope of practice at the hospital. These appointments specify the types of procedures and treatments the medical practitioner is authorised to perform at the hospital, as well as any limitations or restrictions.

The relationship between the hospital and the doctor may be further formalised through a contract or agreement that outlines the terms and conditions of their service arrangement, including compensation, liability, and any other relevant exposures or responsibilities. In most cases, the health service's 'Bylaws' stipulate the obligations and expectations that are conferred upon appointed medical practitioners, and act as the governing guidelines in relation to both clinical practice and professional behaviour standards.

It is important for medical leaders to understand that being credentialed, accredited, or appointed to a private health service requires the medical practitioner to comply with the rules and regulations of the organisation. However, it is not in itself a contractual agreement that the parties enter into and may not confer upon the medical practitioner any right of access to a particular operating list, theatre sessions or ongoing access to practice at the hospital's facilities.

In the Western Australia case of v *Health Solutions 2017*, the court found that the hospital had entered a contract with the applicant upon re-accreditation; however, this only extended so far as to grant *clinical privileges* and did not confer any rights on the practitioner with respect to the allocation of any theatre sessions. The process of credentialing and appointment to a private hospital was described in this case as being akin to 'a ticket that provides entry to the showground (hospital), which does not include the right to ride any particular attraction, i.e. use of theatres/facilities. That latter right must be the subject of a separate commercial agreement.

6.5 Implementing a Credentialing Process in a Private Health Service

Depending on the size and complexity of the private organisation, the credentialing and defining scope of practice for medical practitioner's process may comprise a single credentialing committee, or it may be a multi-step process. Outlined below is one example of a multi-stage system suitable for a moderate to large private health service.

6.5.1 Stage 1: Expression of Interest and Initial Assessment

Specialists may apply or respond to direct invitations or advertisements for appointment. Applications are assessed based on whether there may be an existing or predicted service need or vacancy at the requested hospital locations or services. This stage will involve and impact the planning for and addressing identified service gaps, workforce shortages, and emerging service areas. The initial review should be supported by business development managers and operational Executive Directors, or similar operational leaders, of the private hospital or health service. If on initial assessment, an expression of interest that has been received is deemed a 'good fit' with the facility/organisation based on facility operational and financial capability, the application is progressed to Stage 2.

6.5.2 Stage 2: Health Service Needs Assessment

The second stage focuses on how well the applicant is compatible with or meets the local service needs of the organisation. This type of assessment may often be carried out by the Medical Director based at the facility, who will have a good understanding of the clinical competence and extent of the scope of practice that is needed to be provided at the site. When undertaking this assessment, the applicant's ability to provide the required local services, meet the service productivity and performance targets, and accept the organisation's values and operational policies should be considered. Key elements that may be considered as part of this assessment include:

- A service plan or proposal that is submitted by the applicant, e.g. the primary location they will be basing their private consulting practice, the type of case mix the applicant manages, their activity levels and throughput, and their plans for integrating existing or new consulting rooms.
- Resource availability at the primary location, such as theatre availability, vacant consulting rooms, marketing support, infrastructure modifications, equipment, and appropriately trained support staff.

- Business viability, sustainability, and potential growth of the applicant's business.
- Applicant's availability for providing on-call, follow-up care, and clinical cover arrangements when unavailable.
- Applicant's contribution to education, research, and leadership activities.
- Any existing business arrangements and demonstrated collegiality in working well with other practitioners of the health service.
- Support for the hospital values and expected behaviours.
- Existing commercial or other conflicts of interest with any of the other medical practitioners or services being provided at the health service.
- Alignment with the health service's workforce strategy and succession planning.

If the application is supported at this level it should proceed to a focused clinical review. If the application is not supported, the applicant needs to be informed, offered to withdraw their application, and further progression of the application halted.

6.5.3 Stage 3: Clinical Review – Credentialing

A comprehensive review of the suitability for clinical practice should be undertaken. This may include detailed analysis of the applicant's qualifications, training, experience, complication rates, adverse events, technical competence, clinical judgement, professional capabilities and knowledge, character, and professional suitability. A medical director and/or credentialing committee should undertake the formal assessment at this stage, which also includes the applicant's registration/accreditation status. This assessment may require evidence of completion across the following areas:

(a) Education and formal training:

Formal qualifications accepted by the relevant registration/licensing board.

Speciality Fellowship details with certification of successful completion of advanced training from the relevant college or equivalent.

Diplomas and accredited training programmes in medical skills and advanced practices where relevant.

(b) Previous experience:

Evidence of relevant clinical activity and prior experience in the scope of practice being requested.

Evidence of recent practice in the scope of practice requested, that is attested to by referees and within the curriculum vitae.

(c) Registration/accreditation status:

Evidence of any conditions or limitations imposed by the Medical Board and/or other relevant licensing agency.

Evidence of any conditions, limitations, or investigations relating to accreditation and appointment at other hospitals or health services.

(d) Appropriateness of referees:

Evidence that the referees nominated are able to judge the clinical competence of the procedures requested by the applicant and are able to attest to this based on recent and relevant direct knowledge or observation of the applicant's performance and experience.

Once the suite of required documents has been collated, the application should be referred to a suitably qualified Peer Reviewer, Clinical Reviewer or Committee for consideration. This may comprise one or more senior medical practitioners already credentialed within the private health service who are practicing or have practiced within the same medical speciality as the applicant.

6.5.4 Step 4: Clinical Review – Defining Scope of Practice

The assessment undertaken by the peer/clinical reviewer (suitable senior medical practitioner) should focus on defining the specific scope or extent of the applicant's capacity and skillset. Clinical service alignment should not be considered at this stage of the process as it should already have been performed at Stage 2 so as to remove the peer/clinical reviewer from being required to consider commercial arrangements which could create potential conflicts of interest. Elements that should be considered by the peer/clinical reviewer include the applicant's:

- Quality of care provided through documented outcome indicators, complications rates, and complaints. This may include contribution to established clinical registries.
- Scope of practice competency via evidence from certificates, logbooks, referee reports, etc.
- Clinical suitability for on-call rosters assessed by breadth of recent experience.
- Commitment and ability to participate in audit, teaching, and/or research.
- For reappointments: Prior participation in audit, teaching, and/or research at the organisation.
- Appropriate referee reports.
- Mentor or proctor reports (if applicable).
- The training, experience, judgement, professional capabilities and knowledge, 'Current Fitness' to practice, character, and confidence held in the applicant as a peer.

The peer/clinical reviewer (or committee) will consider the application and define a recommended scope of practice that matches with the applicant's capability and experience. A suitable mentor may be considered for junior or new appointments. A recommendation for approving the delineated scope of clinical practice should then be made to the delegate authorised to appoint medical practitioners to the health service as per its Bylaws (this is commonly the role of the Chief Executive or Chief Medical Officer).

6.5.5 Stage 5: Appointment or Reappointment

If the recommendation is accepted by the delegate, an offer of appointment shall then be made in writing, including any required undertakings and acknowledgements, and the appointment will be effective once it has been signed by the appointee.

If the recommendation is not accepted by the delegate, there may be a 'right of appeal' offered to the applicant. Usually, new (initial) appointment applications will have no rights of appeal.

6.6 Case Study 1: Credentialing Failure

You are the Chief Medical Officer (CMO) of a large hospital system with an auditing and analytics team who monitor and review the clinical outcomes of accredited doctors, with a particular focus on their morbidity and mortality outcomes.

Routine practice involves the team sharing these outcomes with the relevant specialist medical practitioners, to look at identifying any opportunities for improvement, changes in clinical practice, or, with regard to any areas of concerning clinician performance.

While reviewing cases in preparation for an upcoming neurosurgical clinical audit, one of your auditing team members, who also practices within the same hospital as a part-time nurse, identifies a significant outcome in relation to an elective neurosurgery procedure. They advise you that a patient in their mid-50s, whilst undergoing an endovascular cerebral aneurism clipping at the hospital recently, suffered a complication resulting in significant blood loss. The patient appears to have been initially transferred to the ICU post-operatively for stabilisation and subsequently admitted to the rehabilitation unit, to recover from a significant clinical deficit. The prognosis was that there was likely to be gradual improvement, although the likelihood of regaining full function was uncertain.

Your audit team member's concern was that the procedure was undertaken by a neurosurgeon who did not appear to have the appropriate scope of practice (SOP) for undertaking such a complex endovascular neurosurgical procedure.

Within your hospital system, the credentialing process includes a thorough review of clinicians' qualifications, training, and experience, with the additional requirement for those undertaking complex procedures to have undergone further training in the form of 'fellowships' or provide other examples of their experience. Evidence of this via the submission of logbooks outlying case load and outcomes, including complications, was a requirement.

At your hospital, any surgeon undertaking complex neurosurgical procedures is required to have submitted this additional form of evidence of training and experience. Your initial investigation into the credentialing events reveals that this particular neurosurgeon seems to have not applied for the complex procedure she was performing, to be added to their scope list, nor had they presented any evidence of training and experience in this area. Based on this, you proceed to conduct a thorough investigation of all circumstances pertaining to this case.

Your investigation identifies that the details of the complication, including when and how it occurred intra-operatively, had been entered into the clinical record, and that the incident had also been reported via the usual incident management system. However, the initial incident management review seems to have missed identifying the discrepancy of the actual procedure undertaken not being listed in the clinician's SOP. You note that your hospital's surgical bookings process for elective procedures does not have the capability for automatic cross-checking of the procedure listed with the clinician's credentialing and SOP, requiring a manual comparison having to be made between two different systems prior to each case being booked.

It's evident that in this case, the booking was accepted prior to checking that the doctor had an appropriate approved SOP. Had this been identified, the booking would not have been accepted, and a notification of the mismatch would have been sent to your office. Further investigation identifies that the doctor has had some training experience in this procedure at other hospitals and had booked the case in question with a second neurosurgeon who is credentialed at your hospital, to assist him as a co-surgeon. The second doctor in fact does hold the appropriate SOP for the particular procedure at your hospital.

In terms of the credentialing-related clinical governance aspects, the investigation focused on the following areas:

1. Individual Clinician Scope of Practice (SOP) assessment, including a thorough review of procedures, surgical interventions, and admissions over the previous three years undertaken by the clinician. This allowed the extent to which the clinician was working outside her SOP to be mapped, including all hospital-acquired complications and other adverse events that were associated with her other cases.
2. An organisation wide review of the SOPs of all credentialed neurosurgeons, including any other clinicians who were performing the procedure at the hospital, was conducted.
3. A review of other procedures similar in complexity to the index procedure, within neurosurgery was undertaken to confirm none had been performed outside appropriately delineated SOPs.
4. A review of the patient's clinical status was conducted by the local department head to determine treatment options and prognosis.

The neurosurgeon involved in the case was formally advised of the commissioning of the investigation due to a breach of the hospital credentialing and SOP policy, and not permitted to undertake further complex procedures while the investigation was underway. The clinician was requested to provide a number of documents as part of the investigation, including evidence of past training and recent experience in performing procedure at other hospitals. The neurosurgeon was also asked to provide a statement outlining the sequence of events leading to the booking of the case, the decision-making that was involved and whether she had been aware that the procedure was outside her SOP.

Open disclosure (OD) was undertaken to advise the patient and their family of this breach in the clinical governance processes and circumstances that led to the doctor practicing outside their approved SOP.

As a consequence of this incident, the organisation undertook the following actions:

1. Education of relevant senior managers and staff within surgical bookings of the importance of checking each individual clinician's SOP against each procedure prior to them being accepted or progressed.
2. All medical practitioners were reminded of their obligations to practice within their approved SOP and requested to review their listed SOP in the hospital's credentialing system, and if required, apply for any changes to their SOP based on their clinical practice
3. Further investigation as to solutions for integrating booking patient administration software with the credentialing system was flagged as a priority health IT project with a view to enabling automating the cross-referencing processes and avoid manual checks.
4. Clarification that all clinical incidents related to clinical practice routinely trigger a review of the individual clinician's SOP. It was noted that this was not done in this case, and had it not been for subsequent identification by the audit team member in preparation for the audit, it may not have been identified by any other means.
5. As this incident could have occurred across a number of other surgical specialties, a general reminder to all surgical department heads and surgeons as outlined above was issued.
6. The hospital's legal team were advised of the breach of the hospital' credentialing obligations, and potential medico-legal and insurance risk was disclosed.

6.7 Advanced Age Practitioner Credentialing

There has been a long-held expectation and obligation across the healthcare sector for medical leaders to take responsibility in, and be accountable for, identifying and managing predictable risks to patient safety in the delivery of clinical care.

Across the health sector, there continues to be rigorous debate regarding revalidation systems, to ensure continued professional development (CPD) and clinical competence of medical practitioners. The rationale for this has been the well-accepted notion that evidence-based approaches to doctors' continuous professional development drive improvement in their clinical practice and result in better patient outcomes (*Australian Commission on Safety and Quality in Health Care* 2015). This is, of course, notwithstanding the dispute of whether CPD compliance alone is in fact sufficient to assure ongoing medical practitioner clinical competence.

Under the *Health Practitioner Regulation National Law,* in Australia, which governs the operations of the National Boards and Australian Health Practitioner Regulation Agency (AHPRA), there are currently strict requirements for mandating all health services' adherence to ensuring appropriate and recent continuing professional development practices in making decisions related to credentialing, appointment, and reappointment of individual medical practitioners (*Safer Care Victoria, Credentialing and scope of clinical practice for senior medical practitioners policy* 2020).

The Medical Board of Australia (Board) has developed a *Professional Performance Framework* to design and conduct screening and remediation approaches to a number of risk factors identified in literature as markers of poor clinical performance (*Department of Health, Victoria* 2011). Of these, the evidence for age-related risk of poor performance is particularly strong. For practitioners of an advanced age, potential age-related cognitive decline presents a greater level of individual risk with respect to their ability to continue professional practice (*Department of Health, Victoria* 2011). The Medical Board has stated plans to propose requiring targeted screening of practitioners over the age of 70 and above, who are providing clinical care, to have regular health checks and formal peer reviews. These checks are designed to assure patients, individual practitioners, employers, and regulators of doctors' continuing ability to provide safe clinical care. As yet, there are no mandated review requirements for advanced-age practitioners in public or private hospitals in Australia.

Most clinicians will no doubt acknowledge the eventual decline in function, exercise a high level of insight and reflection, and modify their clinical (or non-clinical) practices in response. This is despite the fact that multiple studies looking at cognitive performance data appear to indicate that self-perceived cognitive changes in memory do not in fact align with objectively demonstrated cognitive outcomes (*Giles et al.* 2007; *Knight* 2016; *Partnering for Performance: A performance development and support process for senior medical staff. Melbourne, Victoria* 2010).

While the majority of clinicians practise safely and are suitably self-aware to retire and/or reduce their clinical practice scope at the appropriate point, there is a very small minority of individuals who may be either unaware of their deficits or in denial of them. Guiding medical practitioners through this transition of their careers is perhaps one of the most daunting discussions for medical leaders to undertake in their careers. This is particularly the case for new and junior consultants in the field of medical management.

Medical leaders will face this scenario at a time when a senior doctor is not only confronting their own mortality but is also faced with having to prove their professional functional competence. This creates the potential to generate an emotionally charged situation of extreme sensitivity and hyper-vigilance where the medical practitioner will at all costs be attempting to safeguard their individual sense of self and ego.

Medical leaders charged with ensuring safe clinical practice and the wellbeing of the medical workforce within health services and hospitals must, therefore, approach any discussions with respect to revalidation, credentialing, and scope of clinical practice delineation reviews of these doctors with an abundance of caution and a great deal of empathy. This is particularly important in the private sector, where the advanced-age practitioner is an independently contracted clinician of the health service as opposed to a salaried employee.

6.7.1 Implementing a Governance System

The first step in establishing a system for having appropriately sensitive oversight of advanced age practitioners' safe clinical practice is for medical leaders, including those in the private sector, to bring this issue to the attention of the organisation's peak governance committees. These may be in the form of hospital Medical Advisory Committees or Medical Councils. Given these committees are usually comprised of senior clinicians in advisory roles, they are the ideal platforms for the initial debates, discussions, and challenging of opinions about such an extremely sensitive and crucial problem.

Given the nature of the topic and the absence of national or state guidelines, regulation, or precedence to recommend a directive course of action, the medical leader must be expectant of, and prepared to be faced with, a great deal of inert resistance, or general unwillingness of the committees to readily commit to a position on the issue. However, when presented with the abundance of literature on the topic of age-related functional and cognitive decline, most medical practitioners will agree that it is indeed an issue that is in need of an immediate solution in the interest of ensuring patient safety.

During this initial process of engaging clinicians and hospital leaders to reach some form of consensus on the issue, an important 'tip' for medical leaders driving the issue is to develop and present a ready-made proposal for the group to consider. In other words, the medical leader must be decisive themselves before attempting to get buy-in from others as to the position they are wanting to bring into their health service. Having a ready-made proposal will allow the discussions to then be steered towards the advantages and disadvantages of adopting the position that is proposed.

Experience has proved this technique is far more productive for medical leaders to adopt than merely requesting the committees to provide the answer to the problem from first principles. The medical leader will find that this will also help to circumvent some of the inherent decision-making inertia that will no doubt be observed.

As an example, a position statement necessitating annual 'reviews' for reappointments/re-credentialing of all doctors over the age of 70 may be developed and presented to the peak clinician group for healthy constructive debate. The position will need to be continuously modified in response to feedback from craft (specialist) group consultations, peak credentialing and appointments committees, and other senior clinicians. A comprehensive and thorough process of ongoing consultation is recommended.

The position statement will need to be underpinned by a strong commitment to support a non-discriminatory, individualised, and procedurally fair approach in supporting all advanced age medical practitioners to continue to deliver safe clinical care where possible. Key parameters that are aligned with the organisation's values and by-laws need to then be developed as part of the position statement.

These include consideration of the following attributes of individual medical practitioners:

- Planned volume of clinical activity and/or proposed modifications to scope of clinical practice.
- Annual and total procedural/consulting activity since the start of their first accreditation at the organisation.
- Annual and total procedural/consulting activity external to the organisation.
- Clinical outcomes, including mortality rates, complications, and/or any incident reports.
- Hospital outcomes, including unexpected readmissions, return to theatre rates, and prolonged length of stay.
- Staff/patient feedback and complaints.
- Participation in continuing professional development and/or peer review activities in alignment with the requirements of the specialist medical colleges.

The position statement that is developed should stipulate the frequency with which the above attributes will be reviewed, e.g. at a minimum every 12-18 months for medical practitioners aged 70 years and above.

In observing procedural fairness, an appeals process must also be set up to support any medical practitioners' right to appeal decisions made on the basis of the above recommended parameters. This is in alignment with the initial commitment that was made to ensure a procedurally fair approach and helps strengthen the position.

The next challenge is the practical implementation and impact management of what will be seen as a relatively bold position statement. Consistency, transparency, and fairness of the process, and allowing for consideration of individual and contextual circumstances and respecting the individual and their inherent degrees of sensitivity to the issue is crucial and must be continually upheld. Respect and understanding of senior doctors in each instance is essential, as (in most situations) it may fall to medical leaders who are relatively junior to conduct these difficult discussions and competency assessments.

To aid this and ensure a reliable standard within the system is upheld, a segmented guideline outlining key behavioural, practice, and cognitive components relevant in competence assessments is recommended to be developed. The guidelines should encompass a self-reflective component that the medical practitioner in question would be encouraged to contemplate, as well as a checklist of key points to help the medical leader guide the discussion. Key components of this guideline are outlined in Table 6.1.

Table 6.1 Discussion checklist (self-reflection to be encouraged at each point)

Medical practitioner's planned volume of clinical activity	Does this represent a decrease in activity when compared with recent/current activity levels?
Current and/or intended participation in an on-call roster	What is the plan for managing this?
Intention to modify scope of clinical practice	Reflective capacity
Medical practitioner's annual and total procedural/consulting activity	Within and external to organisation
Clinical outcomes (including mortality rates, complications, incident reports)	Comparisons with colleagues
Hospital outcomes (including unexpected readmissions, return to theatre rates, operating time, and prolonged length of stay)	Comparisons with colleagues/peer organisations
Staff/patient feedback and complaints	Further inquiry as indicated if relevant
Continuing professional development (CPD) plans	Alignment with speciality college CPD requirements
Approach to navigating new/emerging medical advances/clinical practices	Particularly any that may replace/enhance components of their current practice
Intended involvement in teaching and research	Continue and/or modify?
Well-being and health checks	General practitioner support? Medical care support?
Retirement plans	Insight and judgement

6.7.2 The *Art* of the Discussion

Whilst checklists and questionnaires certainly have a place in aiding consistency and comprehensiveness of such discussions, and the medical leader is strongly recommended to adopt these, the true art of engaging doctors in sensitive issues such as this cannot be replaced or overlooked.

This requires a great deal of emotional intelligence and reflective capacity on the part of medical directors/administrators who are facilitating these discussions. He/she must be able to continuously modify and adapt their approach, style of conversation, and demeanour. Careful observation and attention to the body language, tone of voice, unintended posturing, choice of vocabulary, and emotional undertones of the individual being questioned/assessed is a crucial aspect of what will determine the success or failure of this method.

Adequate time and opportunity for the doctors to self-reflect and judge their capacity for themselves must be allowed for during each interaction. Acknowledging any apparent sensitivities from the outset and actively exploring those emotions and/or even reluctance to participate in such discussions will help neutralise tension and unintended emotional bearings. Splitting the discussion into manageable blocks and conducting it over a number of days is another technique that might be preferred by some. This will be particularly useful if any serious concerns are flagged that warrant further examination, which may hinder our ability to reach a mutually agreed outcome with the medical practitioner.

This is an extremely sensitive topic that will undoubtedly lead the medical leader to have difficult conversations with some of their most esteemed and senior medical practitioners. No doubt there will be progressive developments, additional research, and regulatory guidance in this area as well as in the broader medical practitioner revalidation approach across Australia and other nations in the coming years.

6.8 Case Study 2: Aged Practitioner Recredentialing

You are advised by a department director that one of the clinicians within the service, a well-respected and highly considered clinician with an impeccable national and international reputation, has had an increased number of clinical incidents following routine procedures. As a gastroenterologist, the individual has significantly reduced his clinical practice over the last year and now undertakes only colonoscopies and gastroscopies.

Your department director advises that over the last 6 months, he has had three incidents where there have been perforations following colonoscopy. Although on each occasion, the complication has been recognised early, the patients have had the appropriate treatment, and there have been no long-term significant impacts, he is concerned that this senior colleague's rate of clinical incidents is now higher than the benchmark and that this may relate to some issues with performing what is generally considered a routine procedure.

He advises you that, in his view, due to the clinician's age, somewhere in his 'mid-seventies', it is time for the clinician to 'pull up stumps' and either take a long retirement holiday or go onto the teaching and lecture circuit.

The clinician is highly regarded within your organisation, and indeed by yourself, and is seen as the originator of the service in your hospital from the outset many years ago, and the founder of the whole clinical speciality at your hospital.

Whilst it is acknowledged that he has reduced his clinical practice substantially and has done so voluntarily over the last few years, he wishes to 'keep his hand in', and is currently doing so by undertaking only these two procedures. Your enquiries find that he is no longer on the afterhours roster, and when you look at his activity from the last 2 years, his clinical case numbers have reduced, and he is now struggling to fill a procedure list once a month.

You ask your department director for advice, and he states that they had already approached their colleague and discussed the options, and their colleague has replied advising they intend to practice for less than another year, know what they are doing, and has had a 'run of bad luck'. Your director advises they feel uncomfortable pursuing the issue any further due to the reputation of the individual as a senior colleague and believes it is now your responsibility to deal with the issue into the future.

Having an excellent relationship with this senior clinician, you determine to meet with them for a cup of coffee and discussion. At that discussion, you raise the issue of his retirement and the possibility of timing regarding when this may occur. The clinician senses there is an ulterior motive to your request about details of his retirement and bristles at the discussion, and the conversation does not proceed as well as you had intended.

The clinician is so offended by the approach that he advised the Chief Executive and feels that he is under siege, that his reputation is being tarnished, that his contribution to the hospital has been ignored, and that the clinical issues raised are out of proportion to what has actually occurred.

The situation is such that not only is the clinician disengaged, but staff who work with the clinician feel that circumstances have been poorly handled, that, generally, there has been a disrespect and disregard for the clinician and their practice and contribution, and that most importantly, the issue of whether or not they should remain undertaking these procedures has now become secondary to the behaviour and tone of the conversations that have happened to this point.

On reflection, you realise that having an unstructured approach to this individual, and to discuss the circumstances his clinical practice and changes that may be required, has resulted in not only an individual disengagement but a general impact to other staff members and reputational damage to yourself and the hospital.

Aged practitioner reviews need to be considered in context of the clinical circumstances and individual circumstances to ensure that an appropriate approach is followed. You note that there has been disruption in terms of the relationship with the clinician and therefore arrange to meet with the clinician on a second occasion. This time, having prepared for the meeting in a more thorough manner, you open the conversation by asking the clinician what their plans and expectations are into the short and long term.

Having apologised for the manner of the previous conversation, and reassured the clinician that no disrespect was intended, you enable the clinician to discuss that indeed they have been considering retiring. It seems they had noted and had held their own concerns regarding their clinical practice but had felt compelled to continue. He reflects that this is because of wanting to preserve his reputational standing and because often he is asked to provide an expert opinion as the most highly trained and experienced proceduralist in this area.

An open and frank yet structured discussion with the clinician enables the two of you to come up with a plan regarding their retirement and exit from clinical practice, but at the same time recognise and enhance his contribution to the hospital, particularly in education and training of clinicians into the future.

You both note that this speciality now requires specific reporting of both case numbers and outcomes to remain credentialed, and that as a result of the reduction in his clinical practice he would no longer comply with those requirements. This gives him an opportunity to exit from this clinical area with a greater sense of purpose with his reputation intact.

It is evident that over recent years, traditional or longstanding concepts of retirement and changes to work/life balances have significantly been reassessed across many professions, and in several industries and other workplaces senior staff to continue to actively contribute well into their later years.

However, there must be a balance between the potential for ongoing contribution versus the understandable impact of age with regards to dexterity and cognitive function. Therefore, it is imperative that an organisation has a well-structured policy and procedure in terms of how to manage clinicians as they age and a structured process in terms of determining with each individual their plans for transition. This is to ensure that the safety and standard of clinical practice is maintained, and ensure that the professional risks to the clinician in terms of their clinical practice is appropriately managed.

Further Reading

Australian Commission on Safety and Quality in Health Care. Credentialing health practitioners and defining their scope of clinical practice: A guide for managers and practitioners. Sydney: ACSQHC, 2015.

Safer Care Victoria, Credentialing and scope of clinical practice for senior medical practitioners' policy. 2020.

Department of Health, Victoria. Credentialling and defining the scope of clinical practice for medical practitioners in Victorian health services – a policy handbook. 2011.

Rosas V. Physician Credentialing: a guide for physician office staff. 2012.

Giles, Christina W., et al. Health Care Credentialing: A Guide to Innovative Practices. United States, Wolters Kluwer Law & Business, 2007.

Knight, Ellis M. The Handbook for Credentialing Healthcare Providers. United States, 2016.

Partnering for Performance: A performance development and support process for senior medical staff. Melbourne, Victoria. Quality, Safety and Patient Experience Branch, Hospital & Health Service Performance, Victorian Government, Department of Health, April 2010.

Towards revalidation in Australia: a discussion. Joanna M Flynn, Med J Aust 2017;206(1):7–8

Health Practitioner Regulation National Law Act 2009. Accessed via https://www.ahpra.gov.au/About-Ahpra/What-We-Do/Legislation.aspx

Expert Advisory Group on Revalidation Interim report. Medical Board of Australia. 2016.

Building a professional performance framework. Medical Board of Australia. Accessed via https://www.medicalboard.gov.au/registration/professional-performance-framework.aspx

Bieliauskas, LA, Langenecker, S, Graver, C, Lee, HJ, O'Neill, J & Greenfield, LJ 2008, 'Cognitive changes and retirement among senior surgeons (CCRASS): results from the CCRASS Study', J Am Coll Surg, vol.207(1), pp. 69–78; discussion 78–9.

Drag, LL, Bieliauskas, LA, Langenecker, SA & Greenfield, LJ 2010, 'Cognitive functioning, retirement status, and age: results from the Cognitive Changes and Retirement among Senior Surgeons study', J Am Coll Surg, vol.211(3), pp. 303–7.

Lee, HJ, Drag, LL, Bieliauskas, LA, Langenecker, SA, Graver, C, O'Neill, J & Greenfield, L 2009, 'Results from the cognitive changes and retirement among senior surgeons self-report survey', J Am Coll Surg, vol.209(5), pp. 668–71 e2.

Research & Evaluation, incorporating ASERNIP-S Age, performance and revalidation – Report. Royal Australasian College of Surgeons (RACS). 2017

7 Clinical Audit and Outcomes Review in Clinical Governance

A key feature of the clinical governance framework is the collection, review, analysis, and benchmarking of clinical outcome data as part of a comprehensive clinical audit program. This includes the triangulation of audit data with clinical incidents, coding data, and case review. The maturity of a clinical outcome and clinical data monitoring program in a hospital significantly depends on the direction of the board and their review of such data, the importance the executives place on the program achieving meaningful improvement, and the preparedness of clinicians, particularly medical staff, to be active participants. Clinician involvement and engagement in the collation of clinical indicators and outcome data and review of cases through an audit program is a fundamental aspect of achieving improvements in patient care.

Within an employed medical model, the clinical audit can be incorporated into part of the daily clinical activities of clinicians. In a private model, particularly one in which practitioners are remunerated based on providing direct clinical care, clinical audit is usually undertaken in the clinician's own time. Therefore, attendance and participation in such audits are often undertaken early in the day or after routine care is provided.

With the advent of virtual technology in the last few years, audit programs have therefore also increasingly been undertaken in this manner, which has helped to increase attendance. It has, however, also created a set of new issues, including that of maintaining the privacy and confidentiality of sensitive information.

Executives responsible for clinical governance should, where possible, attend clinical audits for a number of reasons.

Firstly, it gives them an understanding of the conduct of the audit. They can be assured that what is being performed meets the professional standards the organisation expects.

Secondly, it provides for an opportunity to confirm that the audit undertaken, discussion of cases, and the findings from audit are rigorous enough to provide opportunities for improvement, and that it is not simply a 'sounding board' with limited review and where opportunities for improvement are not determined.

© The Author(s), under exclusive license to Springer Nature Singapore Pte Ltd. 2026
L. Prado, S. Chandrasiri, *The Practice of Clinical Governance*,
https://doi.org/10.1007/978-981-19-7896-8_7

Thirdly, it gives the opportunity for the executive to query current policies and programs that are in place, to question whether best practice has been followed, and to be assured of the clinical effectiveness of the clinical procedures being provided by the service. It also allows for participants to direct their concerns, for example, regarding resourcing and staffing, directly to the executive, using actual case examples of where deficiencies may have occurred resulting in poor outcomes.

A significant challenge for clinical audit scenarios remains the 'openness' of participants to discuss cases outside their own profession. For example, a clinical audit involving nurses and allied health professionals can prove difficult to arrange, particularly in the private healthcare sector, where specialists may be concerned about potential harm to their reputation, as this could relate directly to their business model and private practice income. Nevertheless, even in these circumstances, the clinical governance leaders should set the tone for open and frank discussion and the importance of having all clinicians present who can then contribute significantly to the audit processes and monitor for meaningful outcomes as a team.

Indeed, clinicians such as nurses and allied health practitioners bring important and alternative perspectives on patient experience, and insights to patient care that the medical staff may not have appreciated.

Clinical audit is also an opportunity for senior practitioners to demonstrate to training specialists, other junior doctors, and clinical staff how to practise professionally, and how to appropriately self assess one's own clinical outcomes. Setting an example and expectation for ongoing learning, by reviewing their own cases as a form of reflective practice can have a significant impact on junior clinicians. Senior practitioners' conduct at the audit and particularly their preparedness to review care, willingness to reflect on decisions they made which could have been different, and their commitment to ongoing improvement, can have a significant positive impact on junior staff and other clinicians.

7.1 Clinical Indicators: Auditing

A rigorous program of clinical audit and review of clinical outcomes is required as a component of clinical governance, and particularly in ensuring that an effective clinical governance framework is in place for preventing unnecessary patient harm. Therefore, as part of the overarching safety and quality system of a health service, establishing a continuous program of clinical audit is recommended.

Criteria for the selection of indicators to be audited, should be determined as part of the clinical governance strategy and approved by the Executive and Board. The indicators that are selected for audit, should be considered carefully and should reflect:

- The capacity of the organisation to monitor them continuously.
- The influence the organisation can have over the performance of the indicator.
- The relevance and impact of the audit on ensuring good clinical governance, how the audited indicators reflect the type and scale of clinical practice improvement required, which can then lead to meaningful practice change.

Standard clinical audit programs commonly include a number of indicators, for example:

- Surgical Safety checklist completion.
- Informed consent completion.
- Completion of documentation of patient assessments such as falls risk, tissue integrity, and nutritional status.
- Completion of discharge summaries.

Following the selection of meaningful clinical indicators, it is important to determine how the indicators will be audited, particularly those indicators that are embedded as part of clinical practice, such as hand hygiene. A key limitation of such clinical audits is that they are, by nature, retrospective and primarily driven by the need to measure compliance, e.g. that policies and procedures of the organisation have been followed by staff.

An example of this is the reviewing of documentation, such as completion of surgical safety check lists following the completion of procedures, to see if they have been completed correctly.

To address this, organisations conduct 'visual' audits: that is real-time auditing of the activity being undertaken by a person experienced in the process, and documenting at that stage whether compliance is occurring. An example of this is a visual audit of the surgical safety checklist and timeout in the operating theatres prior to commencing the procedure.

These two types of audits may result in different outcomes in terms of policy compliance. Visual audits are both time-consuming and resource-intensive compared to 'paper', or 'post activity' audits. However, 'visual' audits are generally more reliable and give a better indication of whether activities are being completed in the correct manner. However, there is a risk of the 'Hawthorne effect' in the case of visual audits, and that compliance by staff is not a true indicator of the actual performance over time.

The relationship of clinical audits to outcome improvement can be problematic to prove. An audit may identify an area of poor compliance, and therefore a program of rectification is then put in place to improve compliance. This is then measured by subsequent audits; however, the impact of that audit may have little bearing with respect to improved patient outcomes.

For example, the auditing of hand hygiene by 'visual' audit can indicate improved compliance with the requirement to perform hand hygiene. However, the relationship of this to a subsequent reduction in hospital acquired infections is more tenuous and difficult to confirm.

Hence, such programs can be difficult to embed as part of clinical practice, as clinicians can struggle to be engaged with what can appear to be a compliance-driven rather than safety-driven process. Nevertheless, clinical audit has a place within the clinical governance framework. The challenge is to identify areas of clinical practice that lend themselves to be audited, and linking the results of audit directly to improvement of patient care and clinical outcomes.

7.2 Clinical Indicators: Development, Monitoring, and Benchmarking

Clinical indicators are data points that can be used to measure the extent to which predetermined targets are achieved, for the purpose of improving outcomes, care processes, and performance of clinical care delivery systems. They can be expressed as numbers, rates, percentages, or averages, and can be either generic across clinical care systems or specific to the disease or speciality area that's being assessed.

Most jurisdictions will have a number of clinical indicators that are routinely monitored and reported to a central 'authority'. In Australia, the *Commission of Safety and Quality in Healthcare (the Commission)* has identified a range of data points that is recommended for use by hospitals to measure the performance of core domains of the clinical care being delivered. These include core hospital-based outcome indicators, such as mortality measures, unplanned readmissions, hospital-acquired complications, patient safety culture measures, patient-reported outcome and experience measures, and clinical condition-based data sets to support monitoring of clinical indicators within clinical care standards.

Clinical indicators should be identified and adopted by individual health services to be reflective of and relevant to their individual patient mix, range of services, and clinical capabilities, from their admitted patient data collections. Monitoring and reporting on these indicators allows for ongoing comparisons of hospital outcomes over time to be made, and for the identification of unwarranted variations that prompt detailed investigations and implementation of changes where required.

National risk-adjustment processes enable for more accurate comparisons between different health services or hospitals, as this takes into account any differences in their patient population demographics. This includes the development of national risk-adjusted coefficients that allow correlations between a particular variable and an outcome, while holding other variables constant (e.g. age, and presence of specific conditions prior to admission).

Stratification of outcomes by hospital peer groups (of similar size and case mix) is another means by which clinical indicators can be compared, and allow for the benchmarking of the outcomes and performance across different hospitals.

Merely reporting on clinical indicators is not a purpose in itself. Two distinct processes need to occur in order for the review of clinical indicators to have any meaningful impact. First, the indicators and trends must be monitored, benchmarked, and reported back to care providers. Second, unsatisfactory scores or any unwarranted clinical or outcome variations, or unwarranted up or down trends, must trigger further detailed investigation and active quality improvement until the indicators are back within acceptable levels.

7.3 Incorporating Clinical Indicators Within Clinical Governance Systems

The board and health service leaders hold responsibility for ensuring that the use of clinical indicators is embedded within clinical governance processes. This includes ensuring that there is strong clinician engagement in the development and selection of indicators that are relevant to the specific clinical speciality. Clinical indicators must also be reviewed, evaluated, and supported by evidence on an ongoing basis to ensure their continued appropriateness and validity.

The role of health leaders in the use of clinical indicators within their organisation's clinical governance framework includes ensuring that processes exist to:

- Monitor any unwarranted variation in practice against expected health outcomes.
- Provide feedback to clinicians on unwarranted variation in practice and health outcomes.
- Review individual service performance against external indicators.
- Support clinicians to take part in clinical reviews of their practice.
- Use information on unwarranted clinical variation to improve safety and quality systems.
- Record and monitor risks identified from unwarranted clinical variation in the risk management system.

7.4 Hospital Mortality Indicators

Hospital mortality indicators (indicators about trends of patient death), such as *hospital-standardised mortality ratios (HSMRs*), allow comparisons between the number of deaths that occurs in a hospital and the number of deaths that were expected to occur, having taken into account hospital and patient-specific characteristics. Hospital mortality indicators are best used as safety and quality screening tools to support clinical governance by flagging potential areas of concern or best practices, not solely as measures of performance on their own.

Deaths in low mortality diagnosis-related groups (DRGs), which report in-hospital deaths for DRGs where the expected mortality rate is less than 0.5%, such as headache, hand procedures, arthroscopy, and *in-hospital mortality rates* for certain conditions, such as acute myocardial infarction, stroke, fractured neck of femur, and pneumonia are also commonly monitored. The four conditions where in-hospital mortality is measured are selected because they are considered 'high morbidity' conditions, which together account for 20% of all hospital deaths, and for which exists standardised models of care, based on clinical evidence. Therefore, reviewing these rates can provide an insight into the performance of specific clinical service lines, as well as a more general indication of patient safety within the organisation. The core hospital-based outcome indicators cited by ACSQHC are listed in Fig. 7.1.

7.5 Hospital-Acquired Complications (HACs)

A hospital-acquired complication (HAC) refers to a complication for which there exists clinical mitigation strategies to reduce the risk of their occurrence, but not necessarily be able to eliminate the risk altogether. Through a process including literature review, and testing with hospitals and clinicians, the ACSQHC has

CHBOI 1 *Hospital standardised mortality ratio (HSMR)*

CHBOI 2 *Death in low-mortality Diagnosis Related Groups (DRGs)*

CHBOI 3 *In-hospital mortality* for:

a) acute myocardial infarction (AMI)

b) stroke

c) fractured neck of femur, and

d) pneumonia

CHBOI 4 *Unplanned/unexpected hospital readmission* of patients discharged following management of:

a) acute myocardial infarction (AMI)

b) knee replacements

c) hip replacements

d) paediatric tonsillectomy and adenoidectomy

Fig. 7.1 ACSQHC core hospital-based outcome indicators list view

determined a list of 16 nationally agreed HACs, with the intention being for clinicians and health leaders to focus on addressing.

These include:

1. Pressure injuries
2. Falls (resulting in fracture or intracranial injury)
3. Healthcare-associated infections
4. Surgical complications (requiring unplanned return to theatre)
5. Unplanned ICU admissions
6. Respiratory complications
7. Venous thromboembolism (VTEs)
8. Renal failure (requiring haemodialysis)
9. Gastrointestinal bleeding
10. Medical complications
11. Delirium
12. Incontinence
13. Endocrine complications
14. Cardiac complications
15. Perineal laceration during delivery
16. Neonatal birth trauma

Figure 7.2 outlines the more comprehensive ACQSHC hospital-acquired complications list. HACs should be monitored at multiple levels within health services, by

Complication	Diagnosis
Pressure injury	• Stage III ulcer • Stage IV ulcer • Unspecified decubitus ulcer and pressure area • Unstageable pressure injury • Suspected deep tissue injury
Falls resulting in fracture or intracranial injury	• Intracranial injury • Fractured neck of femur • Other fractures
Healthcare-associated infection	• Urinary tract infection • Surgical site infection • Pneumonia • Blood stream infection • Infections or inflammatory complications associated with peripheral/central venous catheters • Multi-resistant organism • Infection associated with prosthetics/implantable devices • Gastrointestinal infections • Other high impact infections
Surgical complications requiring unplanned return to theatre	• Post-operative haemorrhage/haematoma requiring transfusion and/or return to theatre • Surgical wound dehiscence • Anastomotic leak • Vascular graft failure • Other surgical complications requiring unplanned return to theatre
Unplanned intensive care unit admission	• Unplanned admission to intensive care unit
Respiratory complications	• Respiratory failure including acute respiratory distress syndrome requiring ventilation • Aspiration pneumonia • Pulmonary oedema
Venous thromboembolism	• Pulmonary embolism • Deep vein thrombosis
Renal failure	• Renal failure requiring haemodialysis or continuous veno-venous haemodialysis

Fig. 7.2 ACQSHC hospital-acquired complications list view

Complication	Diagnosis
Gastrointestinal bleeding	• Gastrointestinal bleeding
Medication complications	• Drug related respiratory complications/depression • Haemorrhagic disorder due to circulating anticoagulants • Movement disorders due to psychotropic medication • Serious alteration to conscious state due to psychotropic medication
Delirium	• Delirium
Incontinence	• Urinary incontinence • Faecal incontinence
Endocrine complications	• Malnutrition • Hypoglycaemia
Cardiac complications	• Heart failure and pulmonary oedema • Arrhythmias • Cardiac arrest • Acute coronary syndrome including unstable angina, STEMI and NSTEMI • Infective endocarditis
Third and fourth degree perineal laceration during delivery	• Third and fourth degree perineal laceration during delivery
Neonatal birth trauma	• Neonatal birth trauma • Hypoxic ischaemic encephalopathy

Fig. 7.2 (continued)

both clinicians and health leaders, and reported to governing bodies such as the Board. Regular monitoring allows the health service to identify any unwarranted variances early, and investigate these in order to implement strategies (such as changes in clinical practice) for reducing the variations. National and peer-hospital rates of HACs are available for external benchmarking to provide context to the interpretation of local health service results.

High or rising rates of HACs indicate that efforts are needed to understand the factors that may be leading to these increases in order to reduce these rates.

Conversely, low and falling rates of HACs can signify success stories, which should be shared amongst clinical teams and leadership groups to encourage and support ongoing quality improvement and maintenance.

7.6 Case Study: Using HSMR in Mortality Reviews

Soon after commencing as the new medical director of a regional hospital in the month of November, you find yourself attending what seem to be quite frequent 'clinical incident review' meetings relating to patient deaths. Many of these have been reported to the coroner due to the patient's death having been 'unexpected' and/or as the cause of the death had been unknown.

During your review, several commonalities between the cases appear to emerge. Some deaths seem to be associated with the sepsis pathway either not having been triggered or not having been followed. Other deaths appear to be related to patients with chronic respiratory and cardiac failure conditions who had been admitted for some variation of an exacerbation of their existing conditions. Further interrogation into each of the cases reveals that the management of Chronic Obstructive Pulmonary Disease (COPD) and Congestive Cardiac Failure (CCF) appears to be quite variable across this health service, both during the emergency department presentation and subsequently during the patient's inpatient stay where they had been admitted to the general medical ward.

This 'cluster' of deaths prompts you to request the hospital's mortality data. You are provided with the HSMR reports including benchmarked figures, that are received by the hospital on a regular basis from an external benchmarking agency the health service subscribes to.

Analysis of these reports show the following:

The HSMR for the June–July 12-month period of the same year is reported at 120, with 50 observed deaths compared to an expected 43 deaths. A figure of 100 is considered 'standard'.

The jurisdiction's HSMR for the same period is reported as being 92, while the HSMR for all benchmarked hospitals is reported as 102.

7.6.1 Case Management

Prior to embarking on managing these findings, it is important to firstly understand the context and significance of the HSMR, particularly in a regional hospital.

7.6.2 HSMR Context and Significance in Clinical Governance

The HSMR is an indicator that acts as a trigger for health services to review any outlier status in their rate of deaths further.

A high HSMR above 100 would not automatically mean there are safety and quality issues. However, it is concerning as it flags a hospital as having 'more deaths than they should be having', particularly if the deaths are considered 'unexpected'.

Whether these unexpected deaths were 'preventable' or not is what is needed to be determined by careful death review on a case-by-case basis.

There are many reasons why an HSMR may be above 100 that may not be indicative of safety and quality failures. These include:

1. Data artefacts—these may be due to coding errors or inconsistencies in the coding practices that exist between different health services.
2. Mortality classification practices—where the criteria used by hospitals to classify a death as expected or unexpected may differ. There could be cases that have been inadvertently incorrectly classified as 'expected' or as 'unexpected'.
3. Medical record documentation errors and the classification of expected deaths being largely based on the accuracy of the medical record—therefore, any errors would lead to an inaccurate calculation of the mortality rate.
4. An unanticipated change in patient mix or services delivered—there may have been an influx of very ill patients that skews the unexpected death rate over a certain period of time.

Whilst identifying all these reasons is important, it is advisable not to automatically assume there is nothing of concern, or that the estimated 'expected death' rates are somehow wrong. The fact that the HSMR has been flagged as an outlier, points to there being something of concern that requires further review. Importantly, the change and trend of the HSMR over months and years should also be seen as a flag. It is important to note that the HSMR is a ratio based on 'total observed deaths' over 'total sum of probability of death'.

If the data that's been reported on the health service's patient admissions and separations was incorrect in any way, then the expected death estimate could indeed be an over or underestimate. However, given that the expected rate is risk-adjusted for patient characteristics, and is a probability measure calculated against death rates of all other similar and non-similar hospitals, it is unlikely that this will be a wrong estimate.

How HSMR calculations are determined is important to clarify, as the HSMR often excludes patient episodes containing palliative care codes, episodes where the condition arose outside the episode of care, patients who self-discharged directly from ED, and patients who left against medical advice. Such situations strengthen the premise that any outlier results are not necessarily simply due to an incorrect estimation of the expected death rate or data inaccuracies.

A key significance of an outlier HSMR, and how this is analysed and monitored, is that it is also an indicator of the maturity and robustness of a health service's clinical governance system. How a healthcare system responds to any variable, and particularly mortality rate variations reflects the following characteristics:

1. A mature and effective clinical governance system, should be able to identify any outlier mortality rates early, for example via a rigorous mortality review system.

2. The level of reluctance/resistance for reporting any outlier findings to the organisation's peak governance committees, including at the board level.
3. The willingness and capability for the findings and data to be shared widely through the clinical governance bodies of the organisation, particularly when such data is indicative of potentially unfavourable outcomes.
4. The capability, capacity, and willingness to initiate an immediate review into investigating the reasons and circumstances around the outlier findings.
5. The ability to critically evaluate and modify processes and systems in response to continuous monitoring of such outlier findings.

7.6.3 Preliminary Analysis of the HSMR

Keeping the above context in mind, we can see that an HSMR of 120 indicates that your hospital is demonstrating a higher-than-standard unexpected death rate when compared to peer hospitals. This is further evident when considering the average HSMR across the jurisdiction where your hospital is located.

As you investigate this, further review of the HSMR report elicits the following findings:

- The difference between the observed deaths and expected deaths equates to seven individual extra deaths over this time.
- The difference in ratios between your hospital's 120 compared to the state-based ratio of 92 shows a ratio difference of 28, which is not a negligible difference and is one which warrants further review.
- The trend graph of the HSMR shows that the unexpected deaths at the hospital appear to have been increasing since June of the previous year. This could point to the cluster of deaths that had been recently observed and indicates the need for these to be investigated further to understand how much of a concern this may be.
- The month-on-month HSMR rates that are presented appear to show that most of these unexpected deaths seem to have occurred within the last 12-month period.
- The variation in the trend of the HSMR over the preceding 5-year period shows there have been three spikes in the HSMR.
- The reports show that almost all the unexpected deaths seem to be arising from emergency department admissions as opposed to elective booked cases, and seem to be occurring more commonly in patients who had been admitted over the weekend (after-hours).
- The 'extra deaths' are seen to be categorised into diseases of the respiratory system, neoplasms, and mental health.

7.6.4 HSMR Interpretation

Based on these review findings, it appears that the HSMR findings point to potential concern in relation to patients presenting to the emergency department of the hospital on weekends.

The interpretation that the findings are more likely to be a cause for concern, as opposed to assuming it is not, is supported by the following:

(a) The variation in the trend of the HSMR over the preceding 5-year period, showing there had been three spikes, tells us that the deaths observed over the recent 12-month period does not appear to be an isolated issue, nor could it have happened 'by chance'. Therefore it is unlikely to be a 'wrong' estimate.
(b) The HSMR ratio in comparison to the jurisdictional ratio showing a difference of 28, is an indication that the difference is likely to be of significance.
(c) As the HSMR trend is observed to be increasing, this is particularly cause for concern, and it is likely that what you have been seeing in the cluster of recent deaths may have been a result of a lack of action with respect to the earlier trend reports. The importance of this interpretation is that, had the findings of these benchmark reports been identified and escalated earlier, perhaps actions could have been put in place to have possibly prevented the recent cluster of deaths from occurring.
(d) Almost all the 'extra' deaths appear to have occurred in the emergency department, and over the weekends. This points to there being a possible systemic issue in this clinical cohort and setting.
(e) On reviewing the trend graphs over a 5-year period, it is noted that there is significant variation month on month in the crude mortality rate as well as the HSMR, where the 'spikes' in mortality numbers are quite frequent and high. Therefore it is again unlikely that this would be due to errors in the estimated expected death rate.
(f) The 'extra deaths' identified are primarily related to diseases of the respiratory and cardiac systems and cardiac metabolic abnormalities, and correlate with the findings of the recent cluster of deaths, as these were commonly in relation to CCF/COPD and Sepsis management. This type of localisation of a high HSMR to one or two disease conditions is indicative of specific cause for concern.

7.6.5 Case Review Action Plan

Having understood the HSMR interpretation in detail, the next step is to extract the relevant medical records of the unexpected deaths for further review. If there is difficulty in local hospital systems correctly identifying the specific cases in question, then all deaths that occurred in the relevant time frame should be reviewed.

These medical records then need to be reviewed in detail by staff or doctors with the appropriate clinical knowledge, with a view to identifying any common root causes.

Meetings with the relevant nursing, medical, and quality leaders should then be convened to share these findings, for the purpose of further understanding any 'on-the-ground' process or systems concerns that may have contributed to them. Meeting early and sharing the findings transparently with these leaders is also key to engaging them in actioning any immediate changes or improvements that may need to be put in place.

The findings, interpretations, and proposed actions should also be tabled at the various relevant clinical meetings, as well as with operational clinical governance committees and board subcommittees for clinical governance.

The mortality review process that is currently in place should be reviewed, including the suitability and adequacy of the expertise available to review deaths at the various levels of the process.

A process for comprehensively analysing HSMR reports as they are received by the hospital, early reporting to Executive and board clinical governance committees, and systems to trigger immediate development and actioning of management plans should be incorporated within the hospital's clinical governance system.

From a clinical care perspective, internal and/or external independent expert reviews into the clinical management of COPD/CCF and sepsis in the emergency department (ED) and the ward should be considered.

Review of the clinical care processes within the ED and ward should focus on the following three key care processes that are commonly associated with high mortality:

1. Recognising clinical deterioration.
2. Escalating concerns regarding clinical deterioration.
3. Clinical handover between the two areas and between teams. It is important that any practice or process improvements that are identified throughout are implemented in a timely manner as they are discovered, rather than waiting until the 'end of the review'.

Finally, it is important that the executive and board are kept informed and prepared for the likelihood that the hospital will likely remain an outlier in HSMR reports for the time being until the impact of change is embedded.

7.7 Clinical Quality Registries in Clinical Governance

Clinical quality registries are usually established by independent organisations that monitor the appropriateness and effectiveness of health care within specific clinical domains or conditions. This is achieved by collaborating with health services to routinely collect, analyse, and report back comparative information on these analyses for the purpose of improving quality and clinical practice.

Clinical registries may collect data retrospectively, currently, or prospectively to systematically collect and analyse data on health outcomes, patient-reported outcomes/experiences, and clinical practice process outcomes for a defined patient population that are risk-adjusted and reported back to the health services for quality improvement.

Well established and successful clinical registries in Australia have organisational governance arrangements, may receive government and/or private funding, and are well coordinated in their function between national, state, and territory governments, relevant clinician cohorts, and key stakeholder groups. Various legislation, regulation, and frameworks relating to the establishment and governance of clinical registries exist in Australia, which includes ensuring relevant data management, data privacy, and confidentiality requirements are met.

Widely used and relatively mature clinical registries that are currently operational in Australia include:

- Australian Rehabilitation Outcomes Centre (AROC)
- Australian Stroke Clinical Registry
- Australian Orthopaedic Association National Joint Replacement Registry (AOANJRR)
- National Cardiac Surgery Database Programme (ANZSCTS)
- Victorian Audit of Surgical Mortality (VASM)
- ANZICS Core Intensive Care Registry
- Prostate Cancer Outcomes Registry (PCOR)
- Consultative Council on Obstetric and Paediatric Mortality (CCOPM)

Registry data can be used by organisations to benchmark their clinical outcomes data. For example, a hospital can benchmark its cardiac surgical outcomes data with those of peer hospitals and compare mortality rates, complications, length of stay, and return to theatre rates. Such benchmarking is invaluable for an organisation if used correctly to drive improvements in patient outcomes.

7.8 Multidisciplinary Meetings

At Multidisciplinary meetings (MDMs) clinicians regularly meet to discuss patients with complex clinical situations to determine the best, most appropriate course of treatment and care. These meetings are cruical to the provision of high-quality care. Examples include patients with cancer, to determine appropriate immunotherapy, chemotherapy, radiotherapy, etc. and structural heart meetings considering care for patients with aortic valve disease determining appropriate medical, surgical or TAVI procedures.

Meeting attendees include physicians and surgeons involved in the discipline, nursing and allied health clinicians, pathology, radiology, and similar providers. By reviewing histology and radiology findings and correlating them to best practice and evidence-based care, clinicians can ensure appropriate treatment plans are developed. In addition, these meetings provide a clinical governance opportunity to measure outcomes against treatment plans, to contribute to audit and clinical registries, and to measure appropriateness, and effectiveness of care. From a governance perspective it is important that the following issues are considered at such meetings:

1. Patient engagement and participation and communication of outcomes.
2. Involvement of primary and community care practitioners and communication of outcomes.
3. Maintaining privacy and confidentiality of discussions.
4. Managing conflicts of interest.
5. Recording of clinical discussions and the appropriate retaining of the records.
6. Contributing to audit and registries.
7. Assessing the actual care given vs the care that was planned.
8. Ensuring that the MDM remains contemporary with regards to best evidence practice.

MDMs require clear governance in terms of the above issues, and this can be achieved with trained, dedicated coordinators using a digital platform to record decisions, which can then be incorporated into other platforms such as the EMR. Appropriate equipment, audio-visual capacity, and video conferencing at these meetings allow for greater participation and engagement. Having all the necessary clinical information available for review at the meeting is key. Good leadership of the meetings ensures that the individual clinical plans are determined, and that coordinators appropriately follow up outstanding actions. From a system governance perspective, hospitals need to ensure that there is a robust process in place that correlates patient admissions for care against the requirement for MDM discussion, so that patients are not admitted, or prescribed care plans without first having their case discussed at an MDM.

Further Reading

Australian Commission on Safety and Quality in Health Care. Using hospital mortality indicators to improve patient care: A guide for Boards and Chief Executives. Sydney. ACSQHC, 2014.

Morrell, Clare, and Harvey, Gill. The Clinical Audit Handbook: Improving the Quality of Health Care. United Kingdom, Baillière Tindall, 1999.

Moorhead, John, and Burgess, Robin. New Principles of Best Practice in Clinical Audit. United Kingdom, CRC Press, 2017.

Clinical Excellence Commission, NSW Health. Guidelines for conducting and Reporting morbidity and mortality/clinical review meetings. 2020.

Dhamija, Bhoresh, et al. Clinical Audit for Doctors and Healthcare Professionals: A Comprehensive Guide to Best Practice as Part of Clinical Governance. United Kingdom, Bpp Learning Media Medical, 2012.

Australian Commission on Safety and Quality in Health Care 2017, National core, hospital-based outcome indicator specification, ACSQHC, Sydney.

H. Wollersheim, R. Hermens, et al. Clinical indicators: development and applications. The journal of Medicine. Netherlands. Accessed via: https://www.njmonline.nl/getpdf.php?id=488

8 Clinical Risk Management

Clinical risk management is a crucial component of healthcare, aimed at proactively identifying, assessing, and mitigating potential hazards that could compromise patient safety and well-being. It involves a systematic approach encompassing various strategies, such as incident reporting, investigation and the implementation of evidence-based protocols. Effective risk management necessitates a collaborative effort amongst all healthcare professionals, and to foster a culture of transparency and continuous improvement. The ultimate goal of clinical risk management is to minimise adverse events, improve patient outcomes, and ensure a safer environment for both patients and staff.

Further, it also plays a vital role in protecting healthcare organisations from potential legal and financial liabilities.

Clinical risk management is the process of identifying, assessing, and managing risks in healthcare services to minimise the likelihood of adverse events and improve patient safety.

It focuses on improving the quality and safety of healthcare services by identifying the circumstances and opportunities that can put patients at risk of harm and acting proactively to prevent or control those risks.

The goal of clinical risk management is to create a culture of safety within healthcare services and to ensure that patients receive high-quality, and safe care.

Clinical risk management is about minimising risks and harm to patients by:

- Identifying what can and frequently does, go wrong during clinical care.
- Understanding the causal and contributing factors that led to adverse events.
- Learning lessons from adverse events and poor outcomes.
- Ensuring action is taken to prevent recurrence.
- Putting systems in place to reduce risks.

© The Author(s), under exclusive license to Springer Nature Singapore Pte Ltd. 2026
L. Prado, S. Chandrasiri, *The Practice of Clinical Governance*,
https://doi.org/10.1007/978-981-19-7896-8_8

Clinical risk management is a key component of a good clinical governance system through which organisations are accountable for continuously improving the quality of their services and safeguarding high standards of care.

Jurisdictions will usually have in place a suite of legislative and regulatory requirements for health care providers to comply with that require specific attention to be placed on the identification and management of risk, especially in terms of clinical practice. As an example, the Departments of Health require all health systems across Australia to comply with specific policy frameworks (*Clinical Governance, Safety & Quality Policy Framework and Risk, Compliance & Audit Policy Framework*) in order to implement and review their clinical risk management systems. Healthcare leaders and staff all hold responsibility to understand and employ risk management in their day-to-day work to provide a safe and secure environment for patients, carers, and staff.

All Australian health services are required to adhere to the systematic risk management processes outlined in the Australian/New Zealand Standard AS/NZS ISO 31000:2018 Standards. Risks are classified according to the *likelihood* of their occurrence and the potential impact of *consequence.*

The health service's risk management framework should define the risk management culture, tolerances, tools to be used, communication and escalation requirements, and reporting processes.

The organisation's *risk management policy* should identify:

- *Who*: is required to report, communicate, and take action.
- *What*: is required to be reported by staff, managers, executives, and governance committees.
- *When*: risks are to be reported and when information is to be distributed to clinicians, staff, executives, and governance committees.
- *Where*: information is stored and communicated.
- *How*: tools and processes are to be used.

Accountabilities and responsibilities held by the governing body, managers, employees, clinicians, contractors, and service providers for risk management should be clearly defined. How the risk management system will be set up and managed will depend on the role, size, and complexity of the organisation. For example, large organisations may have a dedicated risk manager role to oversee the risk management system, while smaller organisations may incorporate responsibilities into existing roles.

Clinical risk management is one component of the more holistic risk management requirements across an organisation. The overarching approach to risk management used across health services is called *Enterprise Risk Management (ERM)* and includes eight domains of risk.

Enterprise Risk Domains

1. Operational risk
2. Clinical (and patient safety) risk

3. Strategic risk
4. Financial risk
5. Human capital risk
6. Legal and regulatory risk
7. Technological risk—cybersecurity
8. Environmental and infrastructure-based hazards

In healthcare, Enterprise Risk Management plans need to be living documents that are frequently updated and improved based on emerging risks, lessons learned, new information, legislative and regulatory updates, and market forces that cause changes within the healthcare system and clinical practice. The organisation's risk appetite and risk tolerance must also be documented, communicated, and regularly reviewed.

8.1 Defining Clinical Risk

Robust risk management processes utilised in clinical settings enable staff and doctors to be actively involved in improving the quality and safety of the clinical services they provide. The effectiveness of managing clinical risk is often highly dependent on the culture of the health service. A culture where patient-centred care is the driving force, ensures that identification and open discussion of mistakes and risks are embedded in the everyday practice of its staff and doctors. A culture of blame creates fear and secrecy, where staff are unlikely to be willing or able to reflect openly and honestly on their clinical practice and processes. Therefore a 'Just Culture' is one that is far more inclusive and likely to create an environment where clinicians are prepared to take responsibility without fear of retribution.

Culture defines the purpose of the health service, what it stands for, what its priorities are, what its values are, how its people are expected to behave and how they interact with each other, as well as how things are done. Culture has the power to influence and define the feelings that staff, doctors, and patients have about the health service, and consequently their actions.

It is the role of healthcare leaders to ensure staff are supported and enabled to confidently discuss any concerns, near misses and mistakes in a just and safe environment where the focus is on improvement. Building a just culture of openness requires processes to be put in place that allow for dedicated, regular time to reflect on clinical incidents and near misses. Leaders need to promote an organisational environment in which a process improvement mentality can thrive, and adequate resources are provided to staff with time for appropriate training, where staff are encouraged to use quality-related tools and techniques on a regular basis. The focus should be on improving processes in the long term and not just patching up protocols and procedures as issues arise.

Effective clinical risk management enables valuable input at every level of the planning cycle of an organisation, from strategic and clinical services planning through to operational plans, departmental plans, and individual clinical program plans. Both clinical risk management and quality improvement should be considered together when determining all operational functions of a health service, including clinical services, capital and infrastructure design and development, equipment procurement, information technology, contractor management, workforce management, financial planning, and occupational health and safety.

The health service may choose to develop a stand-alone clinical risk management plan, but this should then be reflected in its strategic and operational plans. Clinical leaders are responsible for developing and establishing an organisation-wide system that monitors and reports on the safety and quality of patient care and informs any changes in practice.

Clinical risk management involves several key steps:

1. *Identification of Risks*: The first step in clinical risk management is to identify potential risks and hazards in the healthcare environment. This can involve reviewing patient records, conducting risk assessments, and consulting with healthcare providers, consumers and other stakeholders. Further data sources include clinical registry data, clinical incident and audit data, hospital accreditation reports, patient and staff complaints, adverse incidents, quality measures (e.g. surgical site infection surveillance data, hand hygiene compliance data), occupational health & safety incidents and reported hazards or near misses.

Key questions to consider when identifying clinical risks:

- What, when, where, why and how are risks likely to occur, and who might be involved?
- What are the sources/causes of each risk?
- What are the consequences of each risk?
- What are the organisation's internal and external obligations?
- Is there a need for further research into specific risks?
- How reliable is the information?
- Have the right people been involved in the risk identification process?
- Is there scope for benchmarking with peer organisations?

2. *Analysis of Risks*: Once risks have been identified, they must be analysed to determine the likelihood of occurrence and the potential impact on patient safety. This information can then be used to prioritise risks and determine the most appropriate risk management strategies. The level of clinical risk is then defined by the relationship between the consequence and likelihood applicable to the identified risk. A risk rating score is calculated with the corresponding scores in the consequence and likelihood tables multiplied together, i.e. *Risk rating score = consequence x likelihood.*
3. *Development of Risk Management Plans*: Based on the analysis of risks, organisations can develop and implement risk management plans to minimise the likelihood of adverse events and improve patient safety. These plans can involve changes to policies and procedures, staff training, and the implementation of new technologies or systems. A decision should be made with regard the risk treatment options, to:

   (a) Avoid the risk.

(b) Improve risk controls.
(c) Share or transfer the risk.

4. *Monitoring and Evaluation*: Clinical risk management is an ongoing process, and it is important to continuously monitor and evaluate the effectiveness of risk management strategies. This can involve regularly reviewing patient records, conducting risk assessments, and collecting feedback from healthcare providers and patients.
5. *Communication and Collaboration*: Clinical risk management involves effective communication and collaboration between healthcare providers, patients, and other stakeholders. This can help ensure that everyone is aware of potential risks and that risks are managed in a consistent and effective manner.

Clinical risk management is also a critical component of value-based healthcare approaches, as it helps ensure that patients receive high-quality, safe care. By proactively managing risks and continuously improving processes, organisations can enhance patient safety, reduce the likelihood of adverse events, and build trust with their patients and stakeholders.

8.2 Tools for Clinical Risk Management

There are several tools used for risk management, including risk matrices, risk registers, and risk treatment plans. Combinations of risk registers, incident monitoring systems, and complaints managing systems are available as electronic software systems that support the clinical risk management activities of a healthcare organisation.

Risk Matrix A 'Risk Matrix' also known as a probability–impact matrix or a risk heat map, is a tool used to visually represent the likelihood and potential impact (consequence) of potential risks. A typical risk matrix consists of a two-dimensional table with one axis representing the likelihood of the risk occurring and the other axis representing the consequence of the risk (Fig. 8.1).

	Negligible Impact	Minor Impact	Significant Impact	Major Impact	Severe Impact
Highly Likely	Medium	High	Very High	Extreme	Extreme
Likely	Medium	Medium	High	Very High	Extreme
Moderate	Low	Medium	Medium	High	Very High
Unlikely	Very Low	Low	Medium	Medium	High
Rare	Very Low	Very Low	Low	Medium	Medium

Fig. 8.1 Example of a risk matrix showing probability vs impact view

The likelihood of the risk is assessed on a scale from low to high, while the consequence is assessed on a scale from low to high or using a numeric value, such as a dollar amount to reflect the cost impact. Each combination of likelihood and consequence is assigned a risk level or risk rating, which is used to prioritise risk management efforts.

Risk Register A 'Risk Register' is a dynamic document used to record and monitor all identified risks. The risk register usually contains the following information:

1. Risk Description: A brief description of the potential risk and its cause.
2. Risk Category: The risk category is used to group risks by type, such as financial, operational, or strategic (in an enterprise risk register) or such as infection control, medical workforce etc. (in a clinical risk register).
3. Likelihood: An assessment of the likelihood that the risk will occur, typically rated on a scale from low to high.
4. Impact: An assessment of the potential impact of the risk on the organisation, typically rated on a scale from low to high.
5. Risk Owner: The person or team responsible for managing the risk.
6. Mitigation Strategies: A description of the actions that will be taken to reduce the likelihood and/or impact of the risk.
7. Risk Status: An indication of the current status of the risk, such as open, closed, or in progress.
8. Risk Priority: A rating of the risk based on its likelihood and impact, which is used to prioritise risk management efforts.

A healthcare organisation will typically have one risk register with multiple components detailing risk for the various areas in the organisation, including discipline-specific or program-specific clinical areas.

Risk Treatment Plan This is a tool used to identify and outline the steps that will be taken to manage and mitigate a specific risk. The risk treatment plan typically includes the following information:

1. Risk Description: A brief description of the risk that is being treated.
2. Risk Owner: The person or team responsible for managing the risk.
3. Risk Assessment/Risk Rating: An assessment of the likelihood and potential impact of the risk.
4. Risk Treatment Strategies: A description of the specific strategies that will be used to manage and mitigate the risk. This may include risk avoidance, risk reduction, risk sharing, or risk acceptance.
5. Implementation Plan: A plan for implementing the risk treatment strategies, including timelines, resource requirements, and responsibilities.
6. Monitoring and Review: A plan for monitoring the effectiveness of the risk treatment strategies and reviewing the risk assessment periodically to ensure that the risk remains properly managed.

The level of inherent risk (level of risk before treatment/mitigation) should be considered along with the level of residual risk (level of risk after treatment/mitigation), as it is important to monitor the effectiveness of controls on risks that are inherently high.

Each organisation decides on which risks it will report and to what level of management. Some health services may report on all risks with high/extreme consequences or all risks with high/extreme likelihood. Often, only those risks that are deemed unacceptable may need to be reported and treated.

8.3 Case Study: Clinical Risk Management

Your organisation is a complex healthcare group with both acute and rehabilitation hospitals. Within your hospital system, there is a maternity service that provides approximately 3000 deliveries per year. The maternity service is in a purpose-made building located within the heart of a large capital city. It is very popular for providing excellent care to the patients who are referred there and is well supported by the medical and midwifery community.

However, over recent times, the service has struggled in terms of growth in a highly competitive market. Your board has asked for a risk assessment relating to ongoing provision of maternity services as part of the portfolio of clinical services provided by the system.

In undertaking this risk assessment, it is important to ensure that all areas are equally considered and to give a balanced view of the risks to the organisation, including clinical, financial, and reputational. Therefore, to undertake the assessment, you create a team of experienced staff members, including physicians, financial analysts, healthcare executives, and managers who are familiar with clinical service planning and who understand the complexity of maternity services.

To ensure clinician engagement, you also recruit obstetricians, midwives, and paediatricians to help undertake this review. You determine that members of the risk management team should lead the initial conversation, as they are more familiar with the subject matter in terms of risk analysis and how to assist a board in determining what risks exist and how to mitigate those risks, where possible.

The team leader assigned to this task, meets with you early in the review process to indicate their concerns with regards progress of the risk assessment. They advise that the team members are split in terms of motivation and drive, with regards to this review. Some of the clinicians appear more interested in ensuring longevity of the service, demanding change, improvements, and additional resources, and appear to be utilising their involvement in the process to leverage their demands.

Others appear to be concerned that the margin analysis, and revenue cost analysis in particular, does not favour the continuation of maternity service and are approaching the problem with a mindset of discontinuing the service. In view of these challenges, you are determined to provide more detailed guidance to the team with respect to the review that is required.

8.3.1 Addressing Clinical Risk

From a clinical risk assessment perspective, you ask the team to do a deep analysis into the activity of the service over the last three years, including complications, lengths of stay, transfers to special care nurseries and neonatal intensive care, maternal transfer to ICU, and morbidities and mortalities associated with both mothers and neonates. You advise that you require benchmarking with similar organisations both within the jurisdiction and nationally, and where possible, internationally, to look at best practices with regard to clinical care. You specifically ask for a comparison of induction rates and caesarean section rates, and for ensuring that the policies and procedures in place for emergency care, such as emergency caesarean sections, meet recommended national and international guidelines.

You emphasise that you are particularly keen to ensure that cases of clinical deterioration are quickly identified, escalated, and managed appropriately and that the clinical resources in terms of staff experience, training, and an appropriate scope of practice are in place to provide the safest environment for neonates and women. You request an assessment to be made particularly in relation to the fact that the service does not have direct access to an intensive care unit, and that escalation for clinical emergencies is determined by the midwifery team, which requires them to contact on-call staff to come to the hospital.

In view of the complexity of the service, you ask for evidence of training and reskilling in terms of neonatal and maternal resuscitation and if there is team-based scenario training for management in emergency situations in the maternity and neonatal departments.

To assist the team, you suggest that an external team member from a 'like' maternity service from another jurisdiction is brought in to provide expertise, balanced and non-biased opinion with regards to the current status of your service.

8.3.2 Addressing Financial Risk

In view of the competitive market in maternity services and the pressure regarding the management of costs, particularly staffing costs, you request that the team determine whether the market for maternity services is indeed growing, and if so, to identify any financial barriers that may exist for patients to access private services.

You request an assessment of any recent changes in health insurance payments to maternity services, length of stay impacts, changes in caesarean section rates, and the costs for labour, in particular in midwifery services. This is taking into consideration the external context of workforce shortages and a labour market that would favour the employees, as this could see high salary rates and unexpected increases in other costs related to staffing.

With respect to service growth, you ask for an analysis of the potential for expanding service levels at your hospital versus competitors, and for an analysis of market supply and demand concerning the maternity services. You are interested in understanding whether the offering from your hospital remains competitive and is able to meet the current market demand.

8.3.3 Addressing Reputational Risk

You request a review of patient, clinician, and other staff experiences with regards to the maternity services, and for benchmarked data of your organisation's patient experience indicators compared with like organisations. A review of social media and other comparative websites, which provide an indicator of how the service is viewed by the community at large, is also included in your request.

8.3.4 Addressing Staffing Risk

You are critically aware of the importance of adequate staffing for your service being key to sustainability as well as service safety. You acknowledge the difficulties in obtaining sufficient midwifery workforce to ensure provision of a safe, high-quality service. Likewise, you encourage the team to recognise the challenges that may have been involved in retention and succession planning for obstetricians, paediatricians, and anaesthetics.

Of concern, you note that the paediatrician workforce has been, in recent times, less inclined to provide neonatal services without significant financial remuneration and other supports for their practice. The combination of these workforce pressures has made the financial sustainability of the service questionable, with staffing costs now significantly higher than previously budgeted and planned.

In addition, you note with the team that the workforce challenges have resulted in significant reliance on agency and locum staff, who are not committed to your service, whose familiarity with the policies, procedures, and protocols of the service is limited, and whose level of commitment to continuing the service is not to the same degree as those employed by the service.

8.3.5 Addressing Medico-Legal & Insurance Risk

You speak to your health contracting and medical insurance teams. They advise that whilst incidents in the maternity services are few and claims are uncommon, when a claim does occur due to a clinical incident, it may result in a significantly higher financial payment. The medico-legal team advises that the insurance premium for the organisation is substantially higher because of the existence of the maternity service, and in the absence of a maternity service, the premium for insurance would significantly reduce.

In addition, you are advised that maternity service claims remain a risk for a substantial period of time following an incident, due to the nature of the type of claim.

The insurance team notes that it can be difficult to obtain hospital insurance for maternity services in view of the risk of high payouts, which has become more prevalent in recent times, and appears to be consistent with international experience.

The clinical services team advises that the absence of a maternity service will have a significant risk on the remainder of the hospital's services, as maternity services are often the first point of entry and experience for patients and their families with the hospital's other clinical services, as maternity service patients and their families often return to have other care provided by the hospital. They are concerned that changes to the maternity services will have an impact on the IVF and gynaecology services as an unintended consequence in particular, and advise strongly that the maternity services risk assessment should not be done in isolation of both IVF and gynaecology services.

In addition, they advise that women's health in general, such as breast cancer, pelvic floor disorders, and other conditions, may also be impacted by any change made to the maternity services, and that the reputational risk to the organisation of such change would be significant. It is further noted that benchmarking exercises have identified that closure of maternity services usually result in significant community backlash. The reputational impact from a political and community perspective can have considerable negative consequences for the organisation, staff, and clinicians, and this impact can be of high significance from a service access and availability perspective.

This case study identifies the complexity of comprehensive risk assessments in clinical practice, and its multi-faceted impact on clinical governance. By identifying all potential risks of a clinical service: financial, reputational, clinical governance, and staffing, a proper assessment can be made, and the value of safety and quality from a risk assessment perspective should not be understated.

It is insufficient to purely look at the circumstances of safety and quality outcomes in determining the risk of a clinical service, and a balanced and considered review of risk is therefore always required to make informed decisions.

Further Reading

Standards Australia, (2005) Governance, Risk Management and Control Assurance.

Auditor General Victoria, (2004b) Managing Risk Across the Public Sector; Good Practice Guide, Victorian Auditor-General's Office: Melbourne.

Australian Institute of Risk Management, (1997) The profession of risk management, The Australian Institute of Risk Management Journal, 6(1): 5–7.

Standards Australia, (2004) Australian and New Zealand Standard, Risk Management AS/NZS 4360:2004, Council of Standards Australia.

Victorian Managed Insurance Authority, (2008) Risk Management in the Victorian Public Sector: Guide for developing and implementing your risk management framework. VMIA Melbourne.

Victorian Healthcare Association, (2009) Managing clinical risk in primary care: A clinical Risk Management Resource.

Donaldson L. Textbook of Patient Safety and Clinical Risk Management. Germany, Springer International Publishing, 2020.

Carroll, Roberta. Risk Management Handbook for Health Care Organizations: Clinical risk management. United Kingdom, Jossey-Bass, 2011.

Risk Management Handbook for Health Care Organizations. United Kingdom, Wiley, 2009.

Kavaler, Florence, and Alexander, Raymond S. Risk Management in Healthcare Institutions: Limiting Liability and Enhancing Care. United States, Jones & Bartlett Learning, 2014.

9 Medico-Legal Implications of Clinical Governance

Medico-legal implications refer to the legal consequences that may arise from clinical practice, including research. The clinical governance framework plays a critical role in mitigating medico-legal risks associated with clinical practice. Medico-legal issues are complex and are governed by a range of laws and regulations. Healthcare leaders and organisations must ensure that they comply with these laws to avoid legal and regulatory action.

Understanding the interplay between clinical governance and medicolegal frameworks is crucial for fostering a culture of safety, minimising risk, and ensuring ethical and legally sound healthcare delivery. Whilst clinical governance systems aim to improve the safety and quality of care provided to patients and reduce the occurrence of adverse clinical incidents as far as possible, there is a clear intersection with a healthcare organisation's legal obligations and duties that govern the standards of care and responses to adverse incidents. This includes the basis for managing litigation and compensation claims by patients when things go wrong. Therefore, failures in clinical governance will potentially expose individual clinicians as well as the organisation to medicolegal risk and have additional implications on insurance premiums and levels of coverage of the service.

The following elements are key areas where medico-legal implications in the context of clinical governance, can commonly arise in healthcare settings:

Informed Consent Obtaining informed consent from patients or research participants is a legal requirement. A healthcare provider is required to provide sufficient information to a patient to enable them to participate actively in decisions about their care. The information should be provided in a language that the patient understands, taking into account the patient's level of literacy. The clinician has a duty to ensure that patients are properly informed about their condition, the range of treatment options available, and the associated risks before any treatment or intervention is provided.

© The Author(s), under exclusive license to Springer Nature Singapore Pte Ltd. 2026
L. Prado, S. Chandrasiri, *The Practice of Clinical Governance*, https://doi.org/10.1007/978-981-19-7896-8_9

The legal significance of informed consent is that it can act as a defence to claims of negligence. If a patient agrees to a particular treatment, having been made aware that it carries a risk of certain complications, it will be difficult to then successfully claim negligence if that said complication subsequently occurs. This is of course only on the basis that the clinician can demonstrate they had taken reasonable steps to avoid the complication from occurring in their care provision. Clinical Governance Frameworks should encompass policies and processes ensuring that all staff are trained in and always act within the relevant legal framework for obtaining informed consent.

Privacy and Confidentiality Clinicians and medical administrators must comply with data protection laws to ensure that patient information, including the medical record, is managed securely and confidentially. Clinicians have access to sensitive personal information about patients and have a legal and ethical obligation to keep this information confidential, unless the patient consents to disclosure, or disclosure is required by law or is necessary in the public interest.

Clinical governance processes must include safeguards to prevent unauthorised access, disclosure, or misuse of patient information. Data breaches pose a significant medico-legal and regulatory risk for healthcare organisations, and therefore robust processes for monitoring, identifying, and reporting is essential, in particular when clinical data has been exposed and patient confidentiality breached.

Negligence Clinicians have a duty of care to their patients. Medical treatment carries a risk of causing harm that may lead to the patient being even worse than they were before treatment. Even if no treatment is provided (perhaps because the condition was misdiagnosed), this can also be harmful. If a patient comes to harm as a result of a clinician's action or inaction, this may lead to a claim for negligence. Negligence is a claim under law that arises when a person suffers damages or injury as a result of a failure by another person to exercise due care.

In general, to succeed in a negligence claim the patient must establish that the doctor (or other health worker) failed to take the steps that a reasonable doctor would be expected to exercise under the same circumstances; this is known as the 'reasonable person in similar circumstances' test. However, as all medical interventions carry an inherent level of risk, a worsening in the patient's condition after treatment does not always mean that the clinician has been negligent, provided that he or she has exercised due diligence in providing reasonable care.

In cases of medical negligence, the court will also scrutinise whether the appropriate systems of accountability were in place and whether individuals fulfilled their designated responsibilities. Failure to demonstrate this, particularly at a managerial level, can lead to significant liability for the health service. A lack of documented processes, audits, or incident reviews can be interpreted as a failure to exercise due diligence, making the healthcare entity more vulnerable to legal challenges. Further, and as has been outlined in previous chapters, effective clinical governance hinges on the systematic collection and analysis of adverse events and near misses.

Learning from both positive and negative experiences is crucial for continuous improvement. From a medico-legal perspective, thorough incident reporting and root cause analysis are paramount. A lack of documentation or evidence that incidents were investigated and acted upon can be construed in court as a disregard for patient safety and a failure in the duty of care. Conversely, a well-documented system of reporting, analysis, and action plans demonstrates a commitment to learning and improvement, which is viewed favourably by legal bodies.

This highlights the importance of having a robust system for incident reporting, ensuring that all staff are trained and comfortable using it, and that identified issues are systematically addressed. The absence of such systems can create a fertile ground for medico-legal claims, particularly if similar incidents occur repeatedly.

Misconduct Clinicians and researchers must adhere to behavioural guidelines and codes of conduct. Misconduct, such as fabrication or falsification of data, or inappropriate behaviour that places the patient or public at risk, can lead to legal action.

Liability and Vicarious Liability Health services' liability with respect to medical negligence can take two main forms: that of direct liability or vicarious liability. Direct liability arises from a failure of the health service to provide a safe and suitable environment for treatment. Vicarious liability arises from the liability that the health service faces (employer) for the negligent acts of its employees. An employer is responsible not only for their own acts of commission and omission, but also for the negligence of their employees, so long as the act occurs within the course and scope of their employment.

Liability arising from the action of those who are under the supervision of a senior clinician or the ownership of an administrative entity, are also examples of vicarious liability. For the supervising person to be liable, there must be a 'demonstrable' relationship that places one in authority over the other (e.g. consultant specialist and junior doctor). If the clinician who is under the supervision of a senior medical professional causes harm through a medical error, the supervising clinician may be held responsible.

A robust clinical governance framework should actively mitigate risks arising from both direct and vicarious liability. This necessitates clear policies, sufficient resources, and effective supervision structures.

End-of-Life Care The law in Australia and in many other jurisdictions allows for advance care planning, which enables individuals to make decisions about their future healthcare in the event that they are unable to communicate their wishes. The law also provides for the withholding or withdrawal of life-sustaining treatment in certain circumstances. Since the introduction of Voluntary Assisted Dying legislation in some Australian states, as has occurred in a number of countries, mitigating the new and complex levels of medico-legal risk involved in the 'voluntary dying' process needs to be considered from a clinical governance context.

Mental Health The legislation for how mental health conditions are managed in each jurisdiction varies, and healthcare leaders must be across the specifics of the legal requirements, such as involuntary detention, and similar issues that occur in patients with complex mental health conditions. The law in Australia provides for the complexities involved in the care of people with mental illness and sets out the procedures for involuntary detention and treatment of people with severe mental illness who are deemed to pose a risk of harm to themselves or to others. Each state and territory in Australia has its own mental health legislation, and the specific requirements and procedures for involuntary detention and treatment vary. Therefore, the level of medico-legal risk management in this context can be complex and varied, and clinical governance systems within mental health services must consider these carefully.

Insurance Implications Clinicians and healthcare systems usually hold insurance policies for adverse clinical incidents and subsequent medico-legal claims. Individual clinicians' indemnity insurance requirements are between themselves and the provider of the policy. For insurance coverage at the healthcare systems level, the organisation, as an entity may choose to insure themselves or take insurance through external agencies. In any form, the level of insurance coverage and the premiums paid are usually associated with the number of claims made and the quantum of those claims.

In negotiating premiums, hospitals and healthcare systems usually meet with insurers and their brokers to determine the impacts and risk exposures of clinical practice on the insurance policies, and particularly how the clinical governance system and safety and quality program that is in place can help prevent claims in the future.

Importantly, for claims that are already in process, how they are managed is critical to the determination of subsequent premiums. Insurance companies enter and leave the market in healthcare usually based on the quantum of claims and the amount each claim exposes the organisation to.

Healthcare services can find it increasingly difficult to obtain insurance in a market where their medico-legal claims are frequently associated with adverse clinical outcomes. In addition to usual provisions from insurers with respect to clinical services, there are usually additional covers and specifications for what are considered high-risk specialities, e.g. maternity services, where claims in cases of poor clinical outcomes can result in multimillion-dollar payments.

Regardless of how the healthcare organisation is insured for medico-legal claims, the quantum and impact of such claims are directly related to the quality of patient care and the robust clinical governance framework that is in place to prevent harm to patients.

When negotiating with insurers, the health service is usually required to present the clinical governance framework under which it operates. Insurers are usually keen to understand the following areas of clinical governance and how they relate to service delivery:

1. *Appropriate credentialling and appointment to practice of clinicians*: Medicolegally, organisations may be held liable for negligent acts committed by

practitioners who have not been properly credentialed. Insurers require to be assured that the process of clinician appointment, credentialing, and determination of the scope of practice at the healthcare organisation is rigorous and that it ensures that clinicians work only within their designated scopes of practice, and therefore do not risk causing patient harm by working beyond the capabilities of their training, education, and experience. In addition to a process for allocating the scope of practice, insurers require an understanding of the processes the health service has in place to demonstrate ongoing compliance with the scope of practice policies, and that 'scope-creep', and working outside the scope of practice does not occur. Providing assurance through evidence of how the health service ensures compliance with credentialing and clinical practice within delineated scopes of practice, as well as the specific processes the hospital system has in place to respond to any breaches in compliance, is critical.

2. *Policies and Procedures*: The insurers require an understanding of the clinical governance responsibilities that exist within the leadership structure and how ensuring compliance with policy, processes and procedures is undertaken. This includes assurances and evidence of processes that ensure appropriate and applicable standards of care for patients are actually maintained and achieved. This is a fundamental tenet of good clinical governance, and being able to demonstrate to the insurer that policies and processes, such as the provision of deep venous thrombosis prophylaxis to patients undergoing elective surgery, are complied with on a consistent basis, and that these processes are monitored closely, with active programmes of improvement in place where required, to ensure the required outcomes are achieved.

   A lack of clear policies, or the failure to implement them effectively, can leave staff unsure of their responsibilities, weaken organisational accountability, and increase the chance of errors. Medicolegally, a failure to implement and adhere to clinically relevant policies can be interpreted as evidence of negligence.

3. *Incident Management*: Active incident management at the time of an incident and the focus on how the patient and their family are interacted with at the time of an incident can significantly impact whether or not the incident results in a medico-legal claim. A failure to report incidents that occur, as required per jurisdictional regualtions, or a superficial investigation that fails to identify the root causes of the incident, can expose the organisation to reputational damage, civil liability, and potential criminal prosecution. Therefore, insurers prioritise an understanding of the clinical incident management system and processes that are in place in healthcare systems, and request assurance that proactive management of clinical incidents by appropriately trained and experienced staff is undertaken. Insurers assess and expect that the healthcare service has systems to facilitate the highest levels of care and due diligence that can be undertaken, in terms of the chance of reducing harm to patients. This includes examples such as identifying and responding to all clinical needs at the time that they may arise, and that transparent and authentic engagement with the patient and their family in the incident management process is undertaken.

   A failure to adequately implement improvements from clinical incident investigations which results in the recurrence of similar incidents, may result in seri-

ous reputational damage and significant medicolegal risk, including personal risk to the individual healthcare leaders responsible for the implementation of change. In some jurisdictions, this includes the notion of 'industrial manslaughter' in situations of avoidable or preventable death of a patient.
4. *Clinical Audit and Documentation*: A failure to act on identified shortcomings from clinical audits can be seen as evidence of a breach of duty of care, should an adverse incident subsequently occur. Inadequate documentation within the audit process, clinical notes, or incident reports can create significant issues in legal proceedings. Clear, accurate, and contemporaneous records are essential, and any alterations must be appropriately documented and justified.

Risk Management Failing to manage risks adequately, especially when they are known or foreseeable, can be seen as a breach of duty of care and lead to liability claims. Medicolegal exposure can extend to other issues, for example, with equipment maintenance/calibration, staffing deficiencies, environmental hazards and medication errors. A comprehensive risk register, updated regularly, linked to relevant policies, and aligned with the organisation's clinical governance structure is essential. Effective communication of risk information is also critical.

Ineffective clinical governance practice can expose healthcare professionals and organisations to significant legal liability and reputational damage. Therefore, healthcare leaders need to consistently prioritise, implement, and meticulously maintain robust clinical governance frameworks to ensure the highest quality of patient care and mitigate legal risks. Meticulous documentation, consistent adherence to protocols, and a sustained commitment to learning and improvement within clinical governance systems, are the cornerstones of medico-legal protection for healthcare organisations.

Sound clinical governance frameworks, implemented proactively and consistently, are not just an ethical imperative but a legal necessity. Expert understanding of the legal framework, in conjunction with proactive risk mitigation strategies, provides a core foundation for high-performing clinical governance.

Further Reading

Janine McIlwraith, Bill Madden. Healthcare and the Law. Fifth Edition, Thomson Reuters (Professional) Australia, 2010

White, Ben. Health Law in Australia. Australia, Law Book Company of Australasia, 2018.

McDonald, Fiona J., et al. Health Law in Australia. Australia, Thomson Reuters (Professional) Australia, 2014.

Freckelton, Ian R. Disputes and Dilemmas in Health Law. Australia, Federation Press, 2006.

McIlwraith, Janine, and Madden, Bill. Australian Medical Liability. Australia, LexisNexis Butterworths, 2013.

Kerridge, Ian, et al. Ethics and Law for the Health Professions. Australia, Federation Press, 2013.

Clinical Services Planning Within a Clinical Governance Framework 10

Clinical governance is the framework that underpins and ensures services are planned and delivered safely and effectively. It sets the standards for clinical practice, provides guidance on risk management, and helps to ensure that clinical services are delivered in a way that is consistent with the overall goals and objectives of the health service.

Governance and stewardship of health services require a number of planning processes that complement and inform each other in enabling the health service to provide safe, effective, and quality services (clinical care). These include an integration of *strategic planning* (which defines the overarching vision and mission of the health service and abiding values that direct its decision-making), *capital planning* (infrastructure and other capital investments needed to deliver its services), *workforce planning* (the appropriate number and skill mix of clinical workforce that is needed), and *business and operational planning* (the financial and operational resources needed), for delivering services in accordance with, and as specified by, its *clinical services plan*.

Figure 10.1 demonstrates the alignment and overarching influence that clinical governance has with strategic and clinical services planning. This allows the health service to ensure the maintenance, improvement, and alterations to its clinical services planning, is always implemented under the guidance and oversight of a robust clinical governance system.

© The Author(s), under exclusive license to Springer Nature Singapore Pte Ltd. 2026

L. Prado, S. Chandrasiri, *The Practice of Clinical Governance*,
https://doi.org/10.1007/978-981-19-7896-8_10

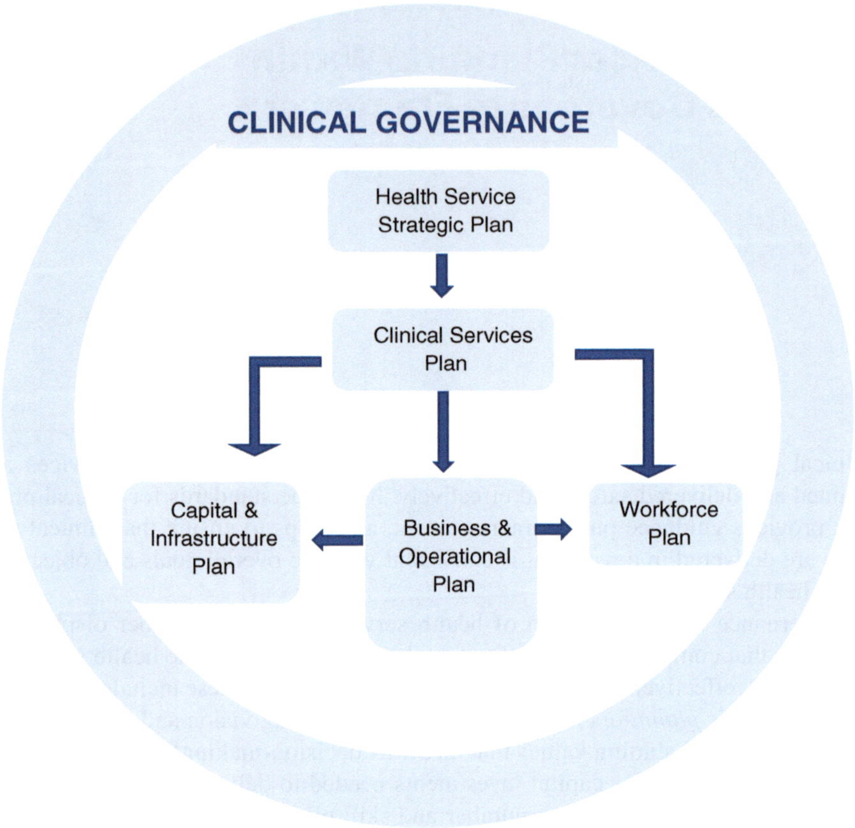

Fig. 10.1 Relationship between clinical governance and clinical service planning (copyright S. Chandrasiri 2023)

10.1 Developing a Clinical Services Plan

The development of a clinical services plan (CSP) must be guided by the key principles that are relevant to the health service and are in alignment with its values. Aligning the CSP to guiding principles such as *evidence-based* approaches, allows for the consideration and investment in emerging clinical practices, research, and technologies that are based on sound evidence to inform future planning. Aligning to guiding principles such as *value* and *outcomes-led* approaches, guides the clinical services plan to be designed and delivered in a way that focuses on and creates value for patients and the organisation, and helps to optimise outcomes for patients.

Flexible and *sustainable* planning ensures continued consideration and responsiveness of the CSP to evolving changes in the healthcare context. A clinical services plan that is developed to meet the health needs of the community, ensures services are designed and delivered in a way that is integrated and coordinated in order to enable easy access and navigation.

Developing a CSP consists of the What, Why, How, Where, and How Much, followed by Monitoring and Evaluation. Figure 10.2 outlines the broader elements of the process and a simple methodology for developing a clinical services plan, whilst Fig. 10.3 explores these elements in more detail.

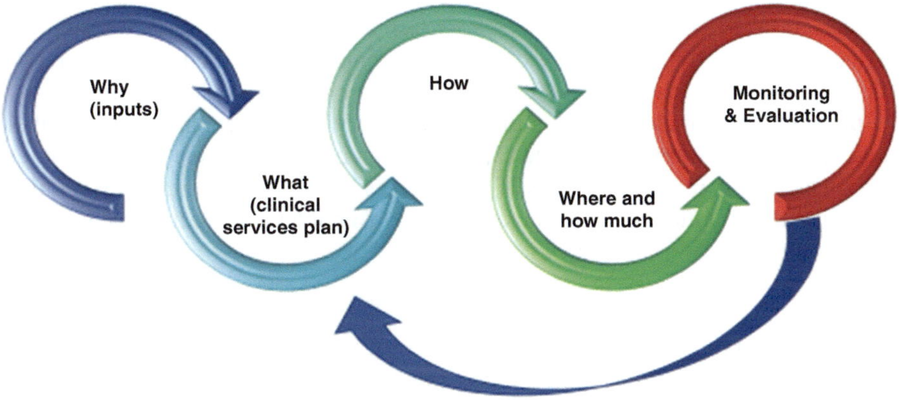

Fig. 10.2 Elements of the clinical services plan development process (copyright S. Chandrasiri 2023)

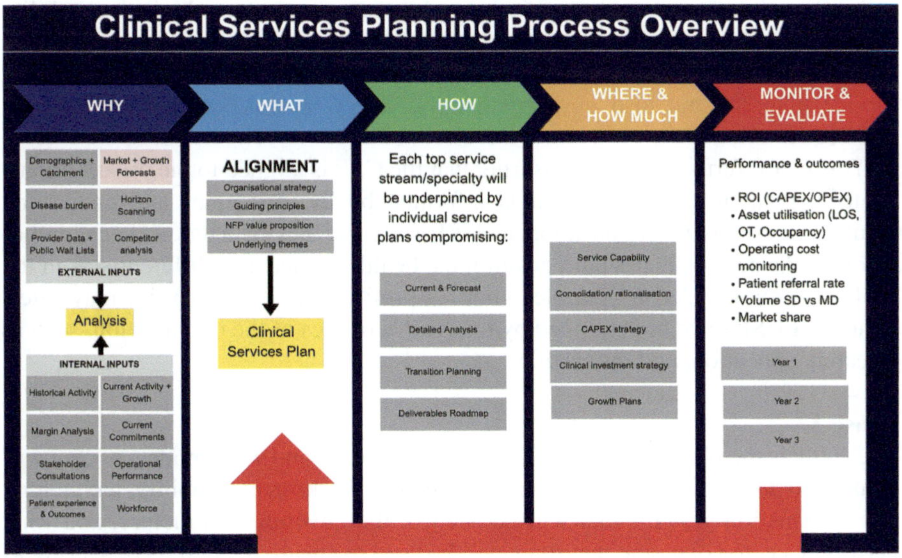

Fig. 10.3 Clinical services plan development methodology framework (copyright S. Chandrasiri 2023)

Phase 1

The *WHY* determines why particular service streams, sub-specialties or models of care are chosen to inform the CSP. This requires an analysis of both external and internal Inputs.

External inputs consider the health service context and healthcare market, including demographics of the catchment area it serves, the disease burden of the population within the catchment, growth forecasts in terms of populations and clinical services market trends, and the impact of competitors in the region (both public and private). It takes a '*horizon scanning*' approach to inform future service delivery. It further considers the risks to the CSP, such as emerging competitors, global risks such as pandemics, changing patient demand, and evolving models of care.

Internal inputs include data on the health service's historical inpatient or outpatient activity, its current workforce capability, outcome and performance measures, and financial and revenue margins of the services currently delivered. This requires extensive consultation with a range of key stakeholders, including patients and doctors.

Phase 2

The clinical services plan is the *WHAT* of the process. It describes the CSP itself and outlines what service streams, sub-specialties or models of care the CSP recommends. It includes a determination of the scope and range of clinical services that are planned to be delivered, e.g. delivering cancer services could include sub-specialised cancer care of breast, ovarian, and pancreatic. This would be dependent on, and require alignment with, health service capability as determined against state and national service capability frameworks that may exist. Clinical capability frameworks define levels of service by describing a set of criteria as minimum requirements for each level of service provision, thus supporting not only clinical service planning but also ensuring quality, safety, access to, and coordination of care.

This phase further involves ensuring that the CSP is aligned to the organisation's strategic plan, is guided by, and is informed by the principles and underlying themes relevant to the organisation, and is based on achieving a unique value proposition and/or factors that would position the health service as a differentiator in the healthcare market. As an example, a not-for-profit (NFP) health service may determine their CSP to be underpinned by the NFP activities of the organisation, such as research, education, and innovation.

Phase 3

The *HOW* is the plan of how the CSP will be delivered and what models of care will be used to deliver it. It considers aspects such as workforce capability, technology and information systems that will be needed, the governance structure, and what performance and outcome measures will be used to ensure the CSP is delivering as intended.

Phase 4

WHERE & HOW MUCH leads to the creation of a *Service Configuration Plan.* This phase determines the locations and volume of services that will be delivered at each site, and over what time frames these will be delivered. Data on activity, margins, demand, and growth forecasts that are specific to each location will need to be analysed as well as current and anticipated disruptors and other forces in ensuring a useful configuration plan

This phase involves an analysis of the return on investment of the existing service configuration and may require recommendations for the consolidation of services, or even rationalisation and planned disinvestment of existing services, in order to free up capacity and capability to deliver the new CSP.

Phase 5

The final phase of CSP development involves the establishment of a monitoring and evaluation roadmap. This allows the implementation of the CSP to be monitored, reviewed, and modified as necessary over periodic time frames. A mixture of both operational performance indicators, such as asset utilisation rates, operating costs, and patient referral rates to each service stream, as well as clinical and quality outcomes, is recommended. These may include a suite of clinical indicators and patient outcomes as determined by and relevant to each speciality area of the CSP, as well as patient experience and satisfaction measures.

10.2 Case Study 1: Closure of a Service

You are an executive in a large private hospital system which consists of a number of facilities ranging from tertiary hospitals with intensive care units, to standalone day procedure units and smaller hospitals with short overnight stays for elective procedures.

In your role as a healthcare executive at this hospital group, you are provided feedback from nursing staff and medical practitioners that some of the procedures undertaken at one of the smaller facilities within the group are inappropriate in terms of complexity, procedure duration, high clinical risk (specifically for select patient cohorts such as paediatrics), and risk of post-operative complications, particularly after hours when there is no medical practitioner available onsite.

You also receive notification from some clinicians, the following additional concerns regarding this site:

1. Inappropriate plastic surgery and cosmetic procedures being undertaken, particularly those involving more than 4–5 hours duration and requiring an overnight stay post-operatively.
2. Concerns regarding inappropriate patient selection, citing cases of patients with BMI over 35 undergoing general anaesthesia and surgical procedures at the hospital.

3. Patients with significant chronic co-morbidities and previous history of anaesthetic risk undergoing complex procedures at the site.
4. Nursing staff highlight concerns regarding post-operative fluid management, blood pressure control, pain management, and the difficulties without an onsite medical practitioner to assist them in decision-making in these areas. They note in particular, patients who have significant cosmetic procedures who may experience large fluid volume shifts in the post-operative period, as being too complex for them to manage without on-site medical input.
5. Nursing staff also raise concerns with respect to patients with significant blood loss who as a consequence require transfusions, being difficult to manage in the absence of a medical practitioner onsite.

To investigate this scenario appropriately you arrange for your team to undertake the standard clinical investigations of each case that had been highlighted by the clinicians as a concern. A review of the cases shows that whilst there had been some difficult post-operative situations, there seems to have been no significant poor patient outcomes. Nevertheless, several critical interventions appear to have been required, including the transfer of patients from the facility to larger inpatient hospitals for ongoing care.

You review the hospital's clinical services plan (CSP) to gain a better understanding of the capacity and capability of the hospital to undertake the procedures that are being booked at this site. To your surprise, you find that the clinical service plan is quite basic and does not in fact consider the service capacity of the hospital, nor the necessary equipment and other requirements that would be standard practice in undertaking the current configuration of complex procedures.

As a result of your initial investigations, you action the following:

1. Request clinicians and anaesthesiologists to advise you on the appropriate clinical risk profile of patients undertaking elective procedures at the facility, particularly accounting for the fact of there being no onsite medical practitioner coverage available after hours, and that any patient requiring significant clinical intervention or escalation of care would be required, by necessity, to be transferred to another facility.
2. Commission the team responsible for clinical analytics to undertake a review of all procedures performed in the facility over the previous 3 years by each practitioner, filtered by speciality and cross-referenced against their individual credentialing and scopes of clinical practice (SOP).
3. Undertake a thorough review of all complications of patients who had been treated in that facility, including any patients who were transferred to another site for ongoing care, patients requiring blood transfusions intra or post-operatively, and those who were readmitted to any other facility post-discharge.
4. Meet with the clinicians providing care and providing the procedures at the site and review their clinical practice, in terms of the range of complexity of cases,

and actively engage with them on available options for managing patients into the future.

5. A thorough clinical governance review identifies that the majority of presenting concerns at this site related to patients undergoing complex cosmetic procedures including total body lifts and similar surgeries where an overnight stay was often required. Due to the nature of their conditions, these patients were at higher risk of anaesthetic problems, particularly due to their BMI. These patients also required transfusions more frequently with difficult-to-manage fluid changes post-operatively. Therefore, as part of your review, an analysis of the skill-set and experience profile of nursing and other clinical and support workforce at this site who are involved in managing complex post-operative patient scenarios is obtained.
6. A review of resuscitation and other clinical equipment, including appropriate monitoring for changes in clinical observations, is also undertaken.
7. You request senior clinicians in each speciality to advise you in relation to any resources and measures that can be considered for immediate implementation at the hospital, to ensure that procedures could be undertaken safely.
8. A financial analysis of the cases that had been undertaken is also conducted in terms of looking at revenue and cost per case, including the cost of patients who required an overnight stay and additional treatment or a higher level of care such as transfusions or transfer to another facility.
9. Clinical risk assessment in terms of the potential for adverse outcomes for patients in this facility is further undertaken, acknowledging the reputational risk if there were significant adverse outcomes, and if a patient was required to be transferred to a larger centre for clinical deterioration or escalation to higher care needs. It is noted that, by the nature of the procedures being undertaken, many of the patients were self-insured, and costs of complications, including treatment for such complications and transfers, were at the patient's own financial risk.
10. A medico-legal risk asessment confirms that the facility was undertaking procedures for which it was potentially not eligible to be covered by its insurance policy, particularly with regard to post-operative complications.
11. A capability assessment is conducted to look at the capability of the hospital site to respond to clinical deterioration and the manner of such responses, in terms of staffing and other resources that are required.

As a consequence of these reviews, it is determined that the hospital's capacity and capability aligns to that of a day procedure unit only, and that no overnight stays should continue. The review also identifies that procedure complexity needs to be modified, and new clinical criteria for patient selection in terms of co-morbidities and anaesthesia risk are required to be developed. Admission criteria that stipulate the appropriate indicators specific for day cases, including type and complexity of procedure, and expected duration of each procedure, are also then developed to ensure that all patients treated are able to be discharged safely on the same day.

The review of inter-hospital and intra-hospital transfer procedures that was undertaken allows for clearer criteria to be determined in identifying patients who, following a procedure and recovery period, may need further treatment. This level of risk stratification and earlier identification enables high risk patients be transferred proactively in anticipation of any sudden clinical deterioration. Additional resources, scheduled training, and equipment is then provided to improve the capacity of the clinicians at the site to be able to appropriately manage the range of complications that are deemed as likely to be expected.

This case study identifies the importance of thorough clinical service planning, including with respect to existing services, in terms of the capacity and capability of a facility, ensuring the appropriate skill mix of its clinicians, and adequate risk assessments of patients and procedures being undertaken. This is critical for healthcare leaders to grasp, in order to ensure that patients are not exposed to unnecessary risk associated with poor service and resource planning, even in scenarios where it may not have been otherwise readily identified or appreciated.

Further Reading

Victorian Department of Health, Health system design, service and infrastructure planning. October 2022.

Eagar, Kathy. Health Planning: Australian Perspectives. United Kingdom, Taylor & Francis, 2020.

WA Health Clinical Services Framework 2014–2024. Australia, Department of Health, 2015.

Queensland Government; Queensland Clinical Services Capability Framework for Public and Licensed Private Health Facilities 2009 (version 3.2). Fact sheet 1 Explanation of service levels.

Thomas, Richard K.. Health Services Planning. United Kingdom, Springer US, 2007.

Safe Introduction of New Technologies 11

Good governance and rigorous oversight of the systems, policies, and processes for safely introducing new technologies and/or new clinical practices in any healthcare setting are of the highest importance. This provides assurance of patient-centred service delivery, clinical safety, and appropriate utilisation of resources within the needs and capabilities of a health service's infrastructure. Particularly in how it aligns with the overarching clinical services plan of the organisation. The introduction of new technologies and new clinical practices in the private healthcare and private hospital sector, can add an extra layer of complexity to this process, given the nuances and unique structures that exist within this sector.

For the purpose of discussion in this chapter, a New Interventional Technology/New Clinical Practice (which we will refer to as NITCP) is defined as any therapeutic intervention and/or clinical practice that is considered by a reasonable body of medical opinion to be significantly different from an existing procedure/clinical practice. In the Australian context, such novel devices must initially be approved and for use and listed on the Australian Register of Therapeutic Goods. It is important that healthcare leaders are aware of the specific legislative and regulatory requirements in their jurisdictions also, for the introduction of new technologies into clinical practice.

11.1 Establishing a System for Governance

Establishing a governance system for the safe introduction of NITCPs ensures that the multiple aspects and their impacts that can be involved, are considered and appropriately assessed. This includes establishing a process by which the organisation will review requests for NITCPs, and specifying who will be accountable for the decision-making. It will further require a process for appeals, a process for evaluating approved NITCPs that are incorporated into clinical practice, and a clear system for how communication will occur with the various relevant stakeholders at each step.

© The Author(s), under exclusive license to Springer Nature Singapore Pte Ltd. 2026

L. Prado, S. Chandrasiri, *The Practice of Clinical Governance*,
https://doi.org/10.1007/978-981-19-7896-8_11

Prior to undertaking the implementation of any system or process of governance, extensive benchmarking with peer organisations of the systems and processes that already exist in the relevant jurisdiction or at a national level, is an important step. Consulting with professional specialty colleges, in addition to literature searches and broad internal stakeholder consultation during the early stages of process development, are also crucial. Multiple forums and consultations with clinicians, medical and clinical directors, operational stakeholders, finance, human resources staff, and medicolegal counsel should be undertaken.

Medical Advisory Councils (and other equivalent departmental group structures) are key appropriate forums for seeking endorsement at the various stages of this process development. Collective forums of hospital medical directors and relevant clinicians can then be convened as required, as they are helpful for refining the more operational considerations, before a newsystem is established.

An extra layer of complexity for establishing governance systems for NITCP reviews in private hospitals exist in this sector. This is due to the nuances of working in an organisation that operates within a private healthcare market. The value proposition of a particular new device/clinical practice being proposed within the private health sector, will have a number of additional variables that come into play when compared with the public health sector. This include considerations such as the value proposition offered to patients from the perspective of what is the best use of their private health insurance, and any out-of-pocket costs that may be incurred in the use of a new device. The financial position, size, clinical activity profile and the financial sustainability of the private organisation within the sector itself, will also feature heavily in the type and scale of system that needs to be put in place at a private organisation when compared to a public organisation.

As an example, most private hospitals may not have 'committees' established that represent the comprehensive cohort of key stakeholders required to consider NITCP applications, as would be usually expected in public hospitals. Most private hospitals will not have junior doctors or salaried doctors to whom evaluation and reporting functions can be assigned. The existing credentialing processes for medical specialists in some of the smaller private hospitals may not be able to incorporate the additional administrative workload of new technology credentialing and ongoing evaluation requirements. Therefore, the capacity to manage a comprehensive system for the review of a NITCP, and monitoring for accurate delineation of the scope of practice for its users, may prove more difficult in these contexts. Business imperatives of individual medical specialists, the impact on their private practices, and impacts on their activity levels at the hospital as a result of bringing in any NITCP, would also factor in these contexts. The common perception and expectation of some private medical specialists that they would automatically be permitted to do any novel procedure they like 'without any red tape' in private hospitals, is both another challenge and nuance that need to be kept in mind.

To address these many challenges and impacts, a multi-pronged and structured process for review is recommended as the framework to be used in developing NITCP governance systems. This includes consideration of any NITCP from multiple perspectives; from an operational and feasibility perspective, an immediate financial perspetive, an overall service sustainability perspective, as well as a clinical safety and efficacy perspective. Additionally, ensuring that the NITCP aligns with the organisation's clinical services plan is also an important component of the assessment to be built in to the process.

The process that is put in place must be adaptable to respond to internal and external market changes, and observed outcomes from the post-implementation evaluations. This allows the organisation to streamline adoption of a NITCP as routine practice or to discontinue the use of any devices/practices that were introduced, with minimal further adverse impact, should it become necessary.

11.1.1 Designing the Governance Process

The following aspects need to be considered in developing a NITCP governance process:

- Registration and approval status with the respective regulatory body.
- Evidence of established or recent use in peer hospitals in the relevant jurisdiction.
- Available body of literature on its use and effects.
- Patient safety aspects including specific impact on patient outcomes and patient experience.
- Clinical effectiveness including comparative performance relative to existing similar technologies/current clinical practices.
- Financial impact including purchase costs, maintenance of any devices, and associated consumables.
- Legal and contractual agreements relating to the procurement and maintenance of equipment and any affiliations with third-party suppliers.
- Impact on existing workflow and hospital operations.
- Availability of appropriate staff including junior doctors, allied health staff, and technicians.
- Credentialing and scope of clinical practice of medical specialists using the device/new clinical practice.
- Impact on payers and funders.
- Patient out-of-pocket costs.
- Any additional training, certification, proctoring, and/or mentoring that may be required.

The process of introduction must also identify any external technicians who may be required to assist in the use of new equipment to conduct the procedure, what their level of credentialing and registration with appropriate professional bodies is required to be, and for whom a clear reporting structure may need to be established.

11.1.2 Hospital-Level Operational Impact

First and foremost, and particularly to allow for those health systems with a somewhat devolved governance structure, the *suitability* for any new NITCP proposal is required to be assessed. This includes the applicant (medical practitioner) and the local governing officer (e.g. a Medical Director) initially discussing the rationale for NITCP introduction and the impact on clinical/safety outcomes that is anticipated. Such discussions will need to be supported by validated literature, discussions with vendors, and with clinicians at other hospitals where the new technology may already have been implemented. The conducting of due diligence to verify independently as to the impact of the new technology is extremely important.

The business development potential for the private hospital and/or for the individual private medical practitioner, will need consideration. Particularly, as there is likely to be flow-on reputational and market impact. The financial costs of purchasing any new equipment, training new staff, ongoing maintenance, and purchase of consumables, compared with the level of private health fund reimbursement rates will need a detailed review to determine the net impact of profitability and financial viability. Other costs associated with the potential impact on existing workflows (e.g. if the use of the new device increases the case time, this will impact theatre utilisation, and there will be a financial impact from the number of cases that will be displaced per day) should also be considered.

A determination as to how the proposed NITCP aligns with the needs and capabilities of the organisation's clinical service plan then adds to the rationale for proceeding with such a proposal. For example, if an organisation's strategic and clinical services plans do not include intentions for growth of their orthopaedic service line, then consideration of any new devices in orthopaedic surgery may not align and may be redundant.

The documentation required at this level should include the following:

- A comprehensive application (a guidance template is provided at the end of this chapter for adapting to your organisation as relevant).
- Current regulatory body approval.
- Literature evidence of clinical effectiveness.
- Description of the conditions and patient cohort that will be impacted.
- Indemnity documentation for the medical practitioner and the organisation.
- Impact assessment as to how integration with (or replacement of) existing workflows of the hospital will be achieved.
- Financial assessment including review of Health Fund contracts and reimbursement rates, particularly as to whether payments will be possible.
- Costing outline inclusive of any direct patient costs and other out-of-pocket costs.

11.1.3 Clinical Effectiveness and Safety Impact

A comprehensive assessment of the clinical impact requires an expert specialist review that would be akin to a clinical departmental or craft group assessment, where relevant senior clinicians of the speciality that the NITCP pertains to are involved. In the private healthcare context, careful consideration must at this point be given to any actual or potential conflicts of interest, as the clinicians involved (those applying for NITCP as well as those considering its assessment) are all independently contracted visiting medical officers with individual commercial and business interests. A key task of the governance body overseeing the NITCP introduction governance system is to ensure that all potential conflicts of interest and/or bias are minimised. Due diligence to determine if private shares are held in any third-party enterprise being considered, and the nature of any professional or personal affiliations and/or competitive business practices between individual medical officers, will also need to be considered.

The clinical reviewer(s) should comparatively evaluate the proposed clinical benefits of a new technology/new clinical practice with equivalent established practice. This is to gain an understanding of the significance and impact of clinical outcomes that will be expected, and to determine a benchmark against which continued utilisation of the technology/new practice can be evaluated. The potential for and severity of adverse patient events, safety concerns, efficacy, and clinical effectiveness measures need to be determined and assessed in light of their acceptability for the patients and the organisation.

11.1.4 Delineation of Scope of Clinical Practice

With the adoption of any new device or new clinical practice, the capability of the individual who will be operating the device or undertaking the clinical practice, requires strict role and scope delineation that is in keeping with the organisation's clinical capability framework. In both the private and public hospital context, this process can usually be aligned to existing credentialing systems and frameworks by which medical practitioners are credentialed and appointed. In the private health sector, this will be under the direction of the health service's regulations (usually the Bylaws), and will include consideration of referee reports, training certificates, level and recency of experience, and professional capability of the individual. A challenge here will be for the credentialing and scope of practice delineations to run concurrently with the process of reviewing and implementing the NITCP.

The credentialing and delineation of scope of clinical practice needs to extend to all other staff involved in the care of the patient as well, including nursing staff, allied health staff, technicians, and junior doctors.

11.1.5 Governance Process Implementation

System level changes and new process implementation require clarity in what is being changed, and should be supported by a suite of documents, as well as training material, to engage the relevant stakeholders in adopting the process. The development of an overarching policy document and supporting protocols outlining the scope and exclusions, clarifying roles and responsibilities, levels of accountability, and dispute resolution processes, is recommended. Further, development of forms and applications with clear criteria for each stage of review will ensure standardisation and consistency, as well as streamlining the process.

A rigorous monitoring and evaluation framework needs to be developed and embedded within the process, for the new technology/new clinical practice to be assessed at ongoing regular intervals. This may be via clinical progress reports or outcome updates, both at an individual case level and at an aggregate level. A process for integrating any recommendations and actions arising from clinical incident reviews can further be embedded as part of the evaluation framework.

11.1.6 Escalation of Concerns

A hallmark of good clinical governance is the ability and responsiveness to the identification, escalation, and management of adverse clinical events. In the same vein, it is crucial to ensure all staff are aware of an organisation's NITCP process and the methods for escalation if there is a breach or concerns with that process. In establishing the system described in this chapter, this escalation process can be incorporated into a hospital's existing incident management system, where notifications of unapproved technology or procedures are reviewed, classified based on potential impact and severity, and responded to by identified staff.

The safe introduction of new interventional technologies and clinical practices to any healthcare setting requires the development and maintenance of a rigorous, sensible and structured multi-step review process.

This is key to ensuring that crucial balance between upholding gold standard and evidence-based medicine, whilst allowing for continuous expansion of existing boundaries through innovation.

Table 11.1 below provides a sample template of an application that can be used by organisations for introducing new technologies.

Table 11.1 Sample template of an application for introducing new technologies

Overview of proposed NITCP		
Name of new interventional technology/clinical practice:		
Category of NITCP:	☐ Prosthesis	☐ Clinical procedure
	☐ Implantable device	☐ Diagnostic technique
	☐ Other (specify):	
Name of individual making the application: Position: Contact details:		
Have you consulted the director of medical services prior to lodging this application?	☐ Yes ☐ No Outcome:	
Classification of NITCP: **Primary site (division/hospital) where the NITCP will be undertaken**	☐ New ☐ Variation to existing intervention/clinical practice ☐ A substitution/ replacement to existing intervention/clinical practice ☐ Other (please specify):	
Has this NITCP been established and/or evaluated elsewhere (nationally and/or internationally)?	☐ Yes ☐ No Please describe:	

(continued)

Table 11.1 (continued)

Overview of proposed NITCP	
Regulatory approval: **Approval from the regulatory authority e.g. in Australia, the Therapeutic Goods Administration (TGA) <u>is required</u> for the introduction of NITCPs.** Please select one of the following: ☐ Australian register of therapeutic goods (ARTG) approved → continue with NITCP application ☐ Specialist access scheme/authorised prescriber approval available → **cease** NITCP application, contact the director of medical services and refer to the hospital's authorised prescriber applications and special access scheme policy ☐ None of the above → **cease** NITCP application, contact the director of medical services	
Does this NITCP have a radiation source?	☐ Yes ☐ No
If yes, does this comply with the hospital's radiation safety protocol?	☐ Yes ☐ No ☐ Unknown
If yes, what compliance activities are required to ensure radiation safety. If currently unknown, please write 'unknown'	
Does this NITCP have a laser?	☐ Yes ☐ No
If yes, please detail compliance activities required to ensure laser safety. If currently unknown, please write 'unknown'	
Please detail compliance activities that are required to ensure electrical safety. If currently unknown, please write 'unknown'	
Have you applied to have this NITCP elsewhere and been refused?	☐ Yes ☐ No
Have you consulted your medical Defence organisation/ indemnity insurance provider?	☐ Yes ☐ No Please specify outcome or provide an explanation:
Scientific evidence Is the proposed NITCP substantiated by high-level scientific evidence in terms of safety (in relation to patients, the individual clinician, colleagues, other staff and the hospital community), efficacy, and clinical effectiveness? ☐ Yes ☐ No If yes (please attach supporting documentation, i.e. RCTs, meta-analyses, systematic reviews) If no → this NITCP must be undertaken within a research setting and/or clinical trial capacity (please contact the research governance unit)	
Clinical impact	
Describe the clinical indication/disease/condition that the proposed NITCP will treat:	
Describe the clinical progression and prognosis of the clinical indication/disease/condition:	
Provide details concerning the incidence and prevalence for the clinical indication/disease/condition in Australia:	
Patient population	
Describe the demographic characteristics of the patient population(s) with the clinical indication/disease/condition (e.g. age range, median and mean, gender, ethnicity, occupation, socio-economic status)?	
What is/are the subgroups of the patient population(s) that will benefit from the proposed NITCP? Please describe the inpatient versus outpatient mix (if applicable):	

(continued)

Table 11.1 (continued)

Overview of proposed NITCP	
Specify the number of adult patients who will receive the proposed NITCP per annum:	
Specify the number of paediatric patients who will receive the proposed NITCP per annum:	
If these numbers are expected to increase over time and/or have a cumulative component due to ongoing follow-up, please specify the predicted numbers of new and follow-up patients by year for 5 years:	
Comparison with existing approach(es) to clinical intervention	
What existing and established interventional procedures/clinical practices is/are used for this clinical indication/disease/condition at your hospital?	
Describe how the proposed NITCP differs from all other available alternatives in current practice, e.g.: • Significant likely clinical advantages over existing treatment (either at this hospital and/or elsewhere): • Potential risks and/or adverse effects from changing to the proposed NITCP	
Opportunities for disinvestment/health service outcomes	
Identify and detail any potential impact on existing services, capital equipment and/or facilities as a result of implementing this NITCP: *Include details about the ongoing ownership of the equipment (hospital or a third party), the contract that will be in place with the procurement team, who will be responsible for ongoing maintenance and servicing reviews. Please provide any written agreements with the technological company and/or procurement team regarding this*	
Patient health outcomes	
What are the patient health outcomes that will be achieved by the proposed NITCP?	
How will these be measured?	
Over what time frame will these be measured?	
Bed utilisation	
Specify whether use of the proposed NITCP will require patients to be managed in:	☐ Intensive care ☐ Multi-day beds ☐ Same day beds
What is the average length of stay per annum for patients receiving the proposed NITCP?	
What bed numbers are required per annum?	
Will this occur within existing capacity? Yes/ no (if no, detail proposed solution)	
How will the introduction of the proposed NITCP affect demand management and access to existing elective and emergency patients?	
Clinical personnel and expertise	
Please specify the type of clinical personnel required to implement the proposed NITCP: *Include any hospital personnel and external clinicians or technicians who may be required either during the procedure or post-procedure*	
Detail the existing clinical personnel and expertise available to implement the proposed NITCP: Detail any discrete and/or additional training requirements for implementing the proposed NITCP: *Include any costs and timeframes associated with this*	

(continued)

Table 11.1 (continued)

Overview of proposed NITCP	
Associated service utilization	
Specify all other services that will be utilised for the proposed NITCP:	☐ Intensive care ☐ Operating theatre ☐ Imaging ☐ Pathology ☐ Outpatients ☐ Other *(specify)*: ____________________
Are these available within existing capacity?	☐ Yes ☐ No → please specify: ____________________
Specify if any clinics and/or wards relevant to each site/setting will be utilised *(pre-admission assessment, inpatient care, and post-discharge care):*	
Implementation documentation	
Please outline the systems for support during the early stages of the introduction of the procedure: Please outline the plan for safe transition from the routine clinical practice (if applicable):	
Patient information and consent forms:	
Is a patient information sheet and consent form attached, including financial consent (please note this is a requirement)?	☐ Yes ☐ No
If no, please explain why not:	
Monitoring and evaluation	
Please comment on each of the following elements that might be considered as part of the monitoring process following the introduction of a NITCP within the clinical setting:	
Learning curve operator(s)	
Credentialing	
Experience	
Quality plan	
Stopping rule	
Other	
Specify an evaluation protocol for the NITCP including performance indicators and defined time points (an evaluation/audit form forms part C of this application)	
Maintenance and security (if applicable)	
Please detail what standard is being used to confirm maintenance and compliance. List the consumables that are required and who will be responsible for procuring and maintaining these. What sterilisation is required and who is responsible for this Detail any software licences that are required, who is responsible for them and under what circumstances will they be novated to the hospital. Detail if the device requires access to the internet through hospital's system and if it requires any cyber-security clearances	
Estimated financial impact	
Please estimate the costs for existing practice (if known): Provide an estimate of all establishment costs for the NITCP (e.g. equipment, capital works, etc.) and how these costs will be met:	
Provide an estimate of all ongoing costs (e.g. consumables, etc.) and how these costs will be met:	
Applicant's Signature	
Signature:	Date: / /

11.2 Case Study 1: Introduction of New Cancer Treatment

As the Director of Medical Services in your organisation, you are approached by the department head of your cancer services, requesting your approval to commence a new treatment for isolated cancer lesions that relate to a new form of innovative therapy which requires implanting a small device at the site of the cancer. He claims that using this new technology will result in reducing the size of the cancer and increasing its likelihood for resection.

The head of department advises you that the technology is well-established overseas, but has not been used before in your country. Nevertheless, he is confident that it is "easy technology to use", and that there should be no concern, as the company that provides the equipment and consumables will provide the equipment console at no charge to the organisation, including the consumables required for the first ten cases. He says the organisation will not incur much expense at all since it will only be required to pay for the ongoing consumables.

When asked, the department head is unable to advise on what the exact cost of the consumables are, but assures you that he is sure that it would be reasonable. If not, he says he is sure that fundraising could support the payments for those, and/or otherwise that the patient could pay the cost of the consumables directly.

You enquire as to the training and experience required by clinicians to undertake this new treatment, and he advises that a representative of the company manufacturing the equipment will be able to attend and train clinicians. In fact, it seems this has already been organised to occur the following week, with the intent being that after a brief introduction to the technology, the representative would remain in the hospital to provide direct proctoring for the clinicians to undertake the therapy.

The department head says that whilst they are a supporter of the therapy, he himself is no longer at the stage of his career for being interested in undertaking this work, but he wants to make sure that it is introduced to the organisation so as to attract more junior clinicians and to retain those they already have.

When you ask the department head to provide greater detail in terms of the risks and benefits, indications for use, and known complications of the therapy, he responds that all that would be a significant amount of work. He does, however, state that he is able to provide papers presented by the company producing the technology, which seems to cite several significant improvements in outcomes for patients. He feels that this should be sufficient, and in view of the fact that the costs will be covered, there really is no negative aspects to introducing the technology as soon as possible.

In managing such a situation, and as covered above, it is important that appropriate governance systems are in place for the introduction of any new technology. Whether or not the new technology has in fact been demonstrated to be effective in other jurisdictions or indeed in an international environment, it is nevertheless important to ensure that your particular healthcare service is able to introduce the technology in a safe and appropriate manner. When assessing new technology, it is not only about determining whether the technology itself has shown benefits for patients or has shown improvements in quality of care, improvements in efficiency, or other areas of improvement. It is also important to determine whether your particular organisation has the capacity and capability to introduce the technology and whether it is able to do so in a manner that is in keeping with the organisation's clinical services plan.

There are many areas of review to be considered. In this case, the department head is asked to ensure that a literature search on the technology including published evidence of journal articles or other forms of clinical peer-reviewed literature is searched for and made available. In addition to the company's own provided literature, it is important to obtain independent information. Where the technology may be so novel that such evidence may yet not be available in peer-reviewed journals, then it is prudent to undertake a review of the sites where the technology has already been introduced, and request this information from the company, so that an independent assessment of the success of the introduction elsewhere could be undertaken.

You advise the department head to make direct contact with organisations that have already introduced the technology and to speak to lead clinicians at those sites. You advise him to specifically ask about any issues experienced with regard to the introduction of the technology, any unexpected or unforeseen consequences observed, and to particularly enquire as to what outcomes had been measured and monitored to date. You request clarity regarding any additional training or skills that would be required by the clinicians and what degree of modifications of credentialing might be necessary to ensure that the appropriate scope of practice is identified for all those involved.

You ask that a suite of clinical indicators and outcome measures be created and/or that if they exist elsewhere, the opportunity to benchmark with like organisations is undertaken. You explain that a comprehensive financial analysis of introducing the new technology is also required because despite the offer for provision of the equipment and initial consumables that has been made, the ongoing consumable costs are no doubt potentially considerable and may have a negative impact on the margin analysis for this particular clinical treatment. Cost considerations are important for viable services, and the consumable costs for this new technology may make the option of introducing this new technology unsustainable in view of these additional costs.

You sense some frustration from your department head initially; however, by discussing with him how these measures relate to ensuring good clinical governance of introducing new technology, you are able to assure him that what you are indeed doing is applying the essential principles of good clinical governance that would lead to the safe introduction of the technology, for an outcome that would be beneficial for both the patients and the clinicians. You also take the opportunity to remind the department head of the many examples of failed introductions of technology in healthcare, and that relying only on the providers of the technology for training, verification of experience, determining outcome measures, and financial advice, is fraught with danger and would be unwise. Using a structured process that is underpinned by good clinical governance when considering the introduction of new technology at an organisation, is therefore an absolute necessity in ensuring both safe patient care and appropriate clinical and operational practice.

Further Reading

McSherry R and Pearce P. Clinical Governance: A guide to implementation for healthcare professionals. Third Edition. 2010.

Chambers, Ruth, et al. Clinical effectiveness and clinical governance made easy. fourth edition. 2007.

Swage T. Clinical Governance in healthcare practice. Second Edition. 2003.

Hospital-Based Health Technology Assessment: The Next Frontier for Health Technology Assessment. Germany, Springer International Publishing.

Anna Flynn and Alison Verhoeven, Deeble Institute Issues Brief. Measuring value in new health technology assessments: a focus on robotic surgery in public hospitals, 2020.

12 Clinical Governance and Value-Based Healthcare

Value-based healthcare focuses on maximising the value delivered to patients, by balancing the quality of care with cost-effectiveness. This approach emphasises outcome measurement and seeks to optimise resource utilisation, while maintaining high clinical standards. The integration of clinical governance principles into a value-based healthcare model is essential for driving improvements in healthcare delivery and ultimately for enhancing patient safety. These concepts are not mutually exclusive but rather interdependent contributors to a robust and patient-centred healthcare system. The core principles of value based healthcare include: prioritising patient-centered outcomes, integrating and coordinating care delivery across sectors and settings, accurately calculating the true costs of care episodes, and aligning payment models to value generation (such as transitioning from fee-for-service to bundled payment models). The most fundamental way that value based care differs from traditional healthcare models, is that unlike fee-for-service, which rewards service volumes, value based care incentivises providers to deliver health outcomes that matter to patients.

12.1 Financial Implications of Clinical Governance

Increasingly, entities that fund healthcare, such as health insurers, funders, and other payers, require healthcare providers to demonstrate clinical governance in practice within their facilities. Most health funding contract negotiations include requirements for healthcare facilities to undertake and demonstrate compliance with hospital-wide accreditation.

Other clinical governance compliance expectations usually include requiring the health service to contribute to clinical registries, demonstrate evidence of undertaking clinical audits, undertake mortality and morbidity reviews, ensure appropriate credentialing and scope of clinical practice (SOCP) delineations for medical

© The Author(s), under exclusive license to Springer Nature Singapore Pte Ltd. 2026
L. Prado, S. Chandrasiri, *The Practice of Clinical Governance*,
https://doi.org/10.1007/978-981-19-7896-8_12

practitioners, undertake patient experience surveys, and show evidence of best-practice clinical incident management protocols.

As health insurance funds usually have access to data such as hospital-acquired complications (HACs) and other outcome data for their members, insurers are increasingly also requiring evidence of performance improvement in hospitals, as part of funding and contract negotiations.

Indeed, recently funders have been requiring evidence of a ‘value-based’ approach to healthcare delivery and have been leveraging outcomes in the form of penalty payments for preventable HACs and other similar contract clauses. These require the health service’s performance to be monitored, measured, and reported to the funders.

It is therefore important that health funding negotiations include the executive or team members responsible for clinical governance at an organisation. Particularly as they can advise the hospital system’s health fund negotiating team with respect to any unrealistic or inappropriate clinical governance outcome measures as KPIs that may be incorporated into contracts by funders. This is especially important if these contractual clauses are in the form of financial penalties and other forms of negative impacts on reimbursement.

Whilst having a shared understanding of clinical outcomes between the health service and health funders is a valuable concept, and indeed can lead to specific improvements in healthcare delivery, it is important that there is also a shared understanding of the direction that such contract negotiations are taking when it involves clinical outcomes.

Consider the following example: A high-performing hospital takes the opportunity to negotiate better reimbursement rates on the basis of its performance in clinical practice, particularly it’s recent reduction in hospital-acquired infections (HAIs).

It is important in this situation that a deep and thorough review of HAIs in terms of what is ‘preventable’ and ‘not preventable’ is understood by all parties first, prior to entering any negotiations and agreements involving any reductions or increases in HAIs. It is also important to be aware that under the guise of clinical governance and outcome measures, such as ‘reducing HAIs’ some health funders may take the opportunity to reduce warranted reimbursement payments (for example for HAIs that may not in fact have been preventable). Therefore, when entering into such negotiations, it is important that experts in clinical governance are advising healthcare negotiating teams and providing the most up-to-date information with respect to how the performance of the organisation can meaningfully be leveraged in funding negotiations.

12.2 Case Study 1: Financial Penalties for Poor Outcomes

During the health fund negotiating process, the health payers’ negotiating team advises your hospital’s contracting team, that they plan to commence a new program of penalties for hospital-acquired complications from the start of the new contracting period.

The health insurer team advises that all hospital-acquired complications, such as infections, falls, and pressure injuries, are no longer going to be funded on a case-by-case basis, since in their opinion such complications should not have occurred in the first place and in their opinion does not reflect good clinical governance.

The hospital's health contracting team determines that if this clause is introduced into the contract, and based on the number of hospital acquired complications that are usually observed at the hospital, it will result in a significant reimbursement penalty to the hospital. The hospital contracting team approaches the clinical executive for assistance to determine to what degree such complications could in fact be preventable, whether they could be reduced in number or prevented altogether, and how the financial impact on the hospital by the new contract requirement could in any way be mitigated.

The clinical executive reviews the contract and notes that the penalty is intended to be applied bluntly for all hospital-acquired complications, regardless of the clinical or patient circumstances involved. It also appears that in managing patients with complex comorbidities, who are inherently at a higher risk of hospital-acquired complications, the hospital would be adversely impacted (from the increased rate of penalties that are likely to be applied to the hospital in caring for the complications that are more likely to occurr in these complex patients).

The team discusses the options with respect to how they should approach the health insurer and the proposed contractual clause. They propose an alternative model to the health fund, where key 'preventable' hospital-acquired complications are selected by the health service and agreed to by both parties are assessed for penalty rate applicability on a case-by-case basis. An example of such a preventable HAC that is provided is an occasion where there has been a failure to administer prophylactic antibiotics in a case of diagnosed surgical infection.

On the advice of the CMO, the team further suggests to the health insurer that the penalties be restricted to a select number of clinical scenarios and in particular to those where an incident investigation has determined that the outcome was indeed preventable.

By negotiating on such rational and patient-centric terms with the health insurer, an agreement is able to be reached that the 'broad brush' approach for penalties cannot possibly be implemented and that the insurer and the hospital would work together towards an outcome-based payment model. The negotiations include financial benefits being provided to the hospital for improved outcomes, for example where there are reductions in hospital-acquired infections, in addition to penalties being applied for preventable HACs after an appropriate review to determine the degree of preventability has occurred.

12.3 Case Study 2: Outsourced Pharmacy Services

A hospital has contracted pharmaceutical services with a large third-party private provider. The services contracted include on-ward pharmacists working with nursing and other clinical staff at the bedside, dispensing medications on discharge, providing imprest drugs throughout all clinical areas, and conducting medication reconciliations on admission.

The pharmacists are directly employed by the third-party provider and work as independent clinicians within the hospital. As part of the contract negotiation between the hospital and the pharmacy provider, it is ensured:

1. That the pharmacists all hold appropriate qualifications and credentialing scope of practice with regards to their performance as a pharmacist on the hospital wards.
2. That there is a clear understanding as to the responsibilities for escalation of any clinical incidents involving the pharmacist, or on occasions where the pharmacist has identified any clinical risks for an individual patient, such as with drug allergies contraindicating the prescription of some medications.
3. Clear provision of medication information at discharge that aligns with the clinical details provided by the ward staff, to ensure there is consistency in the information that is provided to the patient, and that it is provided in a timely manner.
4. Incidents involving pharmacists are notified to team leaders and other physicians in positions of responsibility, so that a joint investigation of clinical incidents can occur and shared learnings and recommendations with regards to any investigation outcomes, are followed through and actioned.

As part of the contract negotiation with the third party, the hospital and the pharmacy provider determine that there will be shared clinical governance projects, such as anti-microbial stewardship, with clear responsibilities and accountabilities for providing expert advice on medication management and tracking of antibiotics used, as well as appropriate reporting to show compliance with best practice guidelines.

An agreement with respect to the third-party provider's involvement in the organisation's clinical governance structures and committees, such as medication safety and medication management committees, is reached. Further, assurance is sought by the hospital that there is to be direct involvement of the third-party provider in providing education, training, as well as being involved in continuous improvement projects at the hospital, in relation to pharmacy and medication safety initiatives.

Agreement on the sharing of accountability for clinical governance, such as in medication-related incident management and in the introduction of new drugs and treatment modalities, is discussed. It is agreed that the third-party provider will manage such situations directly with the hospital, rather than with the hospital's privately contracted medical and nursing practitioners, to ensure that both the quality and safety measures of new treatments are in place, as well as to ensure that the costs of medications are controlled.

During the first 12 months of the partnership, the cost of a medication used in anaesthetics, is observed to substantially increase over 12 months. As part of the clinical governance focused contract that was entered into by the hospital, the pharmacy supplier is required to investigate and work collaboratively together with the hospital, in identifying where and how the cost increase occurred, and to source alternative therapies for practitioners to consider, that were equally effective but less cost inhibitive.

12.4 Value-Based Healthcare

As stated at the start of this chapter, value-based healthcare focuses on maximising the value delivered to patients, by balancing the quality of care with cost-effectiveness. Where clinical governance principles are integrated with value-based models of care, there is potential for significant improvements in healthcare delivery and patient outcomes.

'Value in clinical governance' refers to the way in which an organisation uses a systematic and structured approach to manage the quality, safety, and effectiveness of healthcare services. Value-based care aligns with robust clinical governance for the following reasons:

1. It is realised through improved patient outcomes, reduced healthcare costs, and increased patient satisfaction. By prioritising quality and safety, organisations can build trust with their patients and stakeholders and ultimately enhance their reputation and credibility in the healthcare community.
2. It is a healthcare delivery model that focuses on improving patient outcomes while controlling costs. It aims to provide high-quality care to patients while reducing excess, improving efficiency and promoting better health outcomes.
3. In a value-based system, healthcare providers and payers (such as health insurers) work together to determine the best possible care for each patient based on their individual needs and health conditions. This type of model incentivises healthcare providers to focus on providing the most effective and efficient care for patients, rather than, for example, ordering unnecessary tests and procedures.

The concept of 'value-based care' began in 2006 with Michael Porter and Elizabeth Teisberg's work on redefining the *zero-sum competition* nature of existing healthcare systems, in which gains in one area of the system arise at the expense of another, to that of a positive-sum competition framework, a win–win situation.

The basic premise underlying this concept is that competition in the healthcare market in its current state is set up in a manner that incentivises cost shifting, encourages increasing patient volumes, and favours process compliance as the means by which outcome evaluations occur.

Healthcare systems involve a complex web of providers, funders, and purchasers that are organised primarily around medical specialties. It is a legacy system where fee-for-service payments incentivises the delivery of increasingly higher volumes of services/activities, and outcomes are measured from a process and compliance-driven perspective. In these systems, each hospital or health service often strives to offer as many lines of services as they can, with each healthcare provider then being limited to serving their immediate geographical catchment areas.

What is being proposed with value-based healthcare is a significant shift in mindset to reshape this situation, focusing on generating value for patients by improving clinical and functional outcomes, or reducing costs, or both, over the full cycle of a patient's care.

It suggests generating unrestricted competition within the healthcare market, driven by consolidating health provider experience and expertise at the disease or condition level of the patient. It emphasises generating competition by adopting funding mechanisms that are aligned to support integrated governance structures that deliver cohesive and coordinated care at both the individual patient and the population level. It encourages competition to achieve better results, to improve patient outcomes, to cover a greater degree of geographical reach, and to standardise high performance across regional and national levels, rather than just at the local health service level.

12.4.1 The Need for VBHC

Health systems and services around the world are facing increasing challenges in the equitable delivery of safe, affordable, and high-quality healthcare. These include the following scenarios/challenges:

- Across health services, there is significant unwarranted variation in resource use, resulting in consequent variation in clinical outcomes.
- Payment structures, in most cases, are not applied to treatment options that are evidence-based, which impacts the right treatment not being selected for the right patient.
- There is an increasing shortage of nursing and medical workforce across the world.
- There is an ageing population with a greater and increasing burden of chronic disease, resulting in significant financial costs to health systems.
- There are health inequalities in terms of access across geographical spans, with remote/regional populations having fewer services available.
- There are significant gaps in health outcomes between population groups, for example Indigenous and First Nations Peoples health outcomes.
- Healthcare expenditure becomes increasingly unsustainable, with increased penalty payments being added on for preventable adverse outcomes, such as hospital-acquired complications.

New and emerging disruptors such as robotic surgery, artificial intelligence, precision medicine, and other new technologies continue to increase healthcare expenditure, with evidence as to their effectiveness and cost benefit often lagging or being non-existent.

12.4.2 Implementing Value-Based Healthcare

Implementing value-based healthcare can be a complex process that involves several key steps and the introduction of value-generating strategies to the health system. These include:

1. Understanding and defining a patient population by disease condition or need. One of the first steps in implementing value-based healthcare is to understand the demographics, health status, and care needs of the patient population that is to be served. This helps to inform the development of targetted care pathways and protocols to ensures that the health service is providing care that is tailored to the specific needs of its patients.
2. Building an integrated care team. A value-based healthcare model typically involves a care team that consists of primary care physicians, specialists, nurses, and other healthcare professionals, who work together to provide coordinated, patient-centred care. Building a strong care team is essential for ensuring that patients receive the right care, at the right time, from the right providers.
3. Establishing care pathways and protocols. Care pathways and protocols are key components of value-based healthcare, as they help standardise care delivery and ensures that patients receive consistent, high-quality care. These pathways should be informed by evidence-based best practices and the specific needs of the identified patient population.
4. Defining and measuring outcomes. Ensuring that short- and long-term outcomes which are relevant to patients, and have been co-designed with patients, are collated and measured. This should include clinical outcomes as well as PROMs (patient-reported outcome measures) and PREMs (patient-reported experience measures).
5. Measuring and managing costs. Using acceptable costing methodologies to collect information on the cost of all resources used over an episode of clinical care for a patient. Exploring value-based funding methods such as bundled payments, for example, a bundled payment for the entire patient journey of hospital admission for hip replacement surgery, including the recovery and rehabilitation episode.
6. Implementing data-driven decision-making. Data is a critical component of value-based healthcare, providing information on patient outcomes, quality of care, and resource utilisation. Implementing data-driven decision-making can help the health service continuously improve its performance and ensure that patients receive the best possible care.
7. Engaging patients, clinicians, and other stakeholders. Engaging patients and stakeholders, including health funders and healthcare providers, is essential for building support and buy-in for value-based healthcare initiatives. This can involve educating patients about their care options, involving them in decision-making and empowering them to take an active role in their own health and well-being.

8. Continuously monitoring and evaluating performance. It is important to continuously monitor and evaluate the performance of any value-based healthcare initiatives, to ensure that they are continuing to meet the needs of your patients and are achieving desired outcomes. This can involve using data to track patient outcomes, health service performance, and resource utilisation, and then using this information to identify specific areas for improvement.

Implementing value-based healthcare can be a challenging process, but it has the potential to improve the quality and efficiency of care, enhance patient outcomes, and reduce healthcare costs. By focusing on value and outcomes, health services can create a more sustainable and patient-centred healthcare system.

12.4.3 Enablers for Value-Based Healthcare Systems

Interoperability standards across information technology (IT) platforms and integrated systems for data collection, monitoring, and sharing need to be developed, capable of analysing complex information and deriving valuable insights. Rural and regional IT infrastructure needs to be strengthened and networked. Innovations that increase value need to be actively encouraged and strongly rewarded.

National and state-based policies for generating value-based competition in the areas of funding, performance accountabilities, regulation, legislation, and service planning need to be developed, which incentivises performance and outcomes over volume. They need to enable the alignment and incentivisation of all stakeholders in the health system towards outcome-based funding and pay-for-performance (vs pay for reporting) accountabilities. This, in turn, will help align health provider and health payer goals.

The key stakeholders who are critical to embedding successful transformations in any healthcare system, the clinicians, need to be actively supported to take up leadership roles and to be engaged in leading value-based care initiatives.

12.5 Case Study 3 Integrating VBHC in a Hospital

The first step of any value-based care model application is to segment the patient population being treated, which is the focus of the transformation. In this case study, we explore the scenario of using a value-based care perspective in reviewing the clinical and operational aspects of joint replacements at a private hospital. Firstly a segment of predominantly privately insured patients who presented for elective hip and knee joint replacements was selected as the target group for review.

Existing IT infrastructure and systems were used to conduct a review of all hip and knee replacements that were performed at the health service over the course of the previous calendar year.

Analytics software was utilised to gain clinical and business insights from routinely collected data. Data relating to hospital activity, costs, and revenue were analysed. Surgical activity and clinical outcomes were then analysed. In order to ensure collaboration and data sharing, a governance structure that facilitated this was initially established under the stewardship of an executive-led clinical services planning committee.

Baseline insights were used to elicit the total number of procedures performed over the time period, the total overnight bed days, the average length of stay, and the total revenue (excluding prosthesis costs) over the same time period. This was determined for both hip and knee replacements.

Significant variability was observed in the volume of hip and knee joint replacement procedures across the different hospital sites within the same health service, in terms of the average lengths of stay and in the revenue per day. This level of variability is significant because it can lead to higher costs, inefficiencies in processes, inconsistent standards of service delivery, and poorer clinical outcomes and patient experiences.

A value-based approach would advocate for the co-location of all aspects of care for the particular segment of the patient population being considered, where the care can be delivered by specialised and multidisciplinary teams of clinicians, within what are called Integrated Practice Units.

Using this as the basis, recommendations for consolidating both hip and knee joint replacement procedures at one hospital site (through the organisation's clinical services planning strategy), were proposed as a possible means of reducing this observed variation, improving outcomes and reducing costs.

Another key finding in reviewing this patient segment, was that there seemed to be a variable referral rate to rehabilitation post-hip or knee replacement, across the healthcare service. This was identified as a second priority area to focus on (again by applying a value-based lens) as to how orthopaedic care will need to be delivered in the future.

A second key tenet of value-based care models is ensuring that services are provided through a patient's entire care pathway. This means taking an integrated approach to the delivery of primary, hospital, specialist, and community care needs of the patient, within a centralised and coordinated system, so that medical care is not provided in silos. With respect to orthopaedic surgery, such value-based models can include incentivising (and funding) the 'bundling' of the post-operative rehabilitation care component, with the surgical care component and the inpatient component. This is in recognition of the crucial role that rehabilitation plays in improving patient outcomes and functional capacity post-surgery, and the potential that exists for 'generating value' for both the patient and the health system.

As a result of applying value-based principles, recommendations in the review of the joint replacement service at this hospital group called for a redesign of the acute to rehabilitation transition process for orthopeadic patients across all sites. This process also included having to identify and review the factors that led to unnecessary wait times for a rehab bed, as well as further exploration of local drivers that were leading to delays and bed blocking more generally across the health servcie.

Engaging with the individual surgeons 'one on one', from the outset in this analysis process, was an important action that elicited these crucial insights and assisted in changing behaviours. It is vital that medical practitioners and other front-line clinicians are actively engaged and involved in co-designing any value-based care models as well as in applying any of its concepts, if there is to be any meaningful improvements to clinical service delivery.

By harnessing the concepts of value-based care frameworks to inform the redesign of how orthopaedic services should be delivered in this case, there were a number of early achievements that were able to be realised. These included a measurable reduction in the average length of stay (ALOS) of both hip and knee replacements at this health service, as well as an increase in the percentage of day of surgery admissions, at the start of these patients' care journeys.

Strong leadership at the executive level across the health service, and continuous and authentic engagement of clinicians was important in overcoming organisational inertia and in fostering collaboration and participation amongst the key stakeholders.

VBHC aligns closely with a safety and quality system and clinical governance framework. In a value based healthcare system, high-quality care and improved patient outcomes are rewarded. This then drives the incentives that are necessary for aligning ethical, professional, and financial investments and outcomes. This alignment can be used, as outlined in this case, to meaningfully improve clinical services delivery by focusing the resources and efforts on the areas where clinical care can be improved. Without considerations of financial impact and its alignment with safety and quality, the practical opportunities for significant improvement can be easily missed. Adopting value based healthcare models within robust clinical governance frameworks and systems, is the key to balancing quality, equity and financial sustainability of the healthcare system.

Further Reading

Bloom AL. The funding of private hospitals in Australia. Aust Health Rev. 2002;25(1):19–39. https://doi.org/10.1071/ah020019.

Understanding the Australian Health Care System – E-Book. United Kingdom, Elsevier Health Sciences, 2012.

Thomas Getzen, Health care Economics. Principles and tools for the Health care industry. 2007.

Department of Health and Ageing. Private Health Insurance (Benefit Requirements) Rules 2011.

McSherry R and Pearce P. Clinical Governance: A guide to implementation for healthcare professionals. Third Edition. 2010.

Chambers, Ruth, et al. Clinical effectiveness and clinical governance made easy. Fourth edition. 2007.

Swage T. Clinical Governance in healthcare practice. Second Edition. 2003.

Hospital-Based Health Technology Assessment: The Next Frontier for Health Technology Assessment. Germany, Springer International Publishing.

Anna Flynn and Alison Verhoeven, Deeble Institute Issues Brief. Measuring value in new health technology assessments: a focus on robotic surgery in public hospitals, 2020.

13 Clinical Governance in Research

Clinical governance in research is an essential aspect of ensuring that research studies are conducted ethically, safely, and effectively, and that the results are valid and reliable. Embedding clinical governance in research involves planning and implementing a systematic approach to managing the risks associated with conducting research studies, from the design phase through to the dissemination of results.

Clinical governance principles should be reflected in all aspects and at all phases of any research that is undertaken. This includes the following stages:

Ethics approval: All research studies involving human participants must be reviewed and approved by an ethics committee to ensure that they meet ethical standards for research.

Protocol development: Researchers must develop a detailed protocol outlining the research question, study design, methods, and procedures that will be followed throughout the study.

Risk assessment: Researchers must identify and manage the risks associated with conducting the study, including risks to participants, researchers, and the broader community.

Data management: Researchers must manage and store study data securely, to ensure that it is accurate, complete, and accessible when needed.

Quality assurance: Researchers must conduct quality assurance checks throughout the study to ensure that data is being collected and analysed correctly, and that the study is being conducted according to the approved protocol.

Reporting and dissemination: Researchers must report their findings accurately and transparently and disseminate their results to relevant stakeholders, such as participants, funders, and policymakers.

Clinical governance in research ensures that the principles, requirements, and standards of research are appropriately rigorous to ensure the protection of research participants, to uphold the safety and quality of the research conducted, and to

© The Author(s), under exclusive license to Springer Nature Singapore Pte Ltd. 2026

L. Prado, S. Chandrasiri, *The Practice of Clinical Governance*,
https://doi.org/10.1007/978-981-19-7896-8_13

ensure privacy and confidentiality aspects are upheld. It further acts to safeguard financial probity, compliance with legal and regulatory requirements, ensures adequate risk management, and that appropriate monitoring and evaluation strategies are in place. In addition, it acts to strengthen and promote a good research culture and practice within the healthcare service.

Healthcare organisations should ensure that their procedures, policies, and other documents that guide good research governance, conduct, and management are open, transparent, and available to members of the community.

Whilst clinical governance requirements in the delivery of clinical services are increasingly well known, and the criticality of patient safety and quality of care in clinical service provision is generally well understood, there is an additional complexity when bringing clinical governance into the realm of research, noting that research involving patients, is usually governed by the research entities overseeing and authorising the programs and participants.

Within healthcare systems undertaking research, there is often significant complexity with regards to ensuring clinical governance of the research conducted, particularly with regard to ensuring the safety and protections of the research participants. The reason for this is that in healthcare systems, much of the research undertaken is in the form of clinical trials, or similar research, that impacts on the clinical care of persons who would normally be patients of the health service, and who have consented to participate in the research as part of an experimental component of their medical treatment.

13.1 Clinical Trials Governance

A clinical trial is any research study that prospectively assigns participants or groups to one or more health-related interventions to evaluate its effects on health outcomes, and may involve treatments, procedures, medical devices, experimental drugs, biological products, or health-related service changes.

Clinical trials governance is often integrated within the larger corporate and clinical governance frameworks of health service organisations and clinical trial sites. It ensures that everyone involved, including frontline clinical trial investigators undertaking clinical trials, and members of governing bodies such as health service boards, is accountable to patients and the community for assuring that the delivery of clinical trials within their service is of high quality, is integrated into practical clinical care, and is continuously improving. The role of clinical leaders, and more specifically leaders of clinical trial services, is to ensure and support a culture of responsible research conduct within their organisations and to actively take part in the development of systems that enable and give priority to high-quality clinical trial service provision. Clinical leaders would be expected to engage with managers (both clinical and non-clinical) regarding the quality of clinical trial service provision through defined and delegated roles and functions, as part of the clinical trial workforce. This may include responsibilities for implementing strategic direction, managing the operations of a clinical trials governance system, reporting on the quality and effectiveness of the research governance system, and implementing the organisation's clinical trial culture of high-quality service provision.

In Australia, clinical trials are delivered by teams of clinical trial investigators, where both clinical and non-clinical staff work in partnership with trial sponsors, regulators, trial participants, consumers, patients, their families, and carers. Clinical trials are delivered in both public and private health service organisations, including at trial sites ranging from sole proprietorships to large statutory corporations and public companies. The National Safety and Quality Healthcare Standards (NSQHS) specify the actions that a health service organisation needs to meet to develop and ensure systems for good clinical trials governance. It is mandatory for all Australian hospitals and day procedure services to be assessed through an independent accreditation process to determine whether they have implemented the NSQHS Standards with regard to clinical trials governance.

Clinical trials are important as they have the potential to provide early access to innovative treatments and interventions for patients, and to improve the overall standard of medical care provided in Australian hospitals through their translation into practice.

Participation in a clinical trial for a patient of the healthcare system usually involves the patient being enrolled to receive new or experimental therapies or treatment modalities, investigations, or diagnostic processes. They are usually enrolled directly by their treating clinician, or on referral by their treating clinician to another clinician who is undertaking the clinical trial (often as the principal investigator). Therefore, when a clinical trial is conducted within the healthcare system where the patient is admitted to receive clinical care, there are additional responsibilities on the system and health leaders with regards to ensuring that the safety and quality of care provided is not inadvertently or adversely impacted by their participation in the trial. In larger organisations, this area of accountability usually sits with dedicated research governance units.

Research governance requires that an individual's consent to participate in research is well documented, that criteria for inclusion into research projects have been specified, and that confirmation has been made that the participant has met those criteria in order to be eligible to participate. From a patient perspective, however, participating in a study such as a clinical trial would often appear to be not that different compared to the standard therapy they would expect to receive. They rightly hold therefore, the same set of expectations as they would hold if admitted as a 'normal patient': i.e. that the facility will continue to provide safe, high-quality care to them.

Indeed, clinical trials are often undertaken in the same clinical area as where standard treatments are delivered and, in fact, often alongside patients who may be receiving the standard treatment, and not uncommonly from the same clinician. In such circumstances, it is important that those responsible for clinical governance in the facility works closely with the research governance unit to ensure there is a shared understanding of the responsibilities for patients who are undertaking research studies at the facility.

A number of key aspects need to be specifically considered in ensuring there is good clinical governance in place for research studies to be conducted. It's prudent to note that the research studies are often conducted within research centres that also provide unique forms of therapy and treatments. Additionally, research studies are often collaborative and therefore maybe provided by healthcare organisations, universities, and other external bodies, such as pharmaceutical companies, in partnership with the health facility.

The following are important foundational aspects of clinical governance of research that healthcare leaders should be familiar with:

1. Ensuring that all researchers who are conducting studies have been appropriately credentialed to the healthcare facility to undertake both the research and the clinical care that is involved. This includes ensuring that the scope of practice (SOP) in realation to the research, particularly if it involves new and innovative diagnostic and therapeutic techniques, is clearly articulated in addition to the scope of clinical practice (SOCP) they may require in providing the care itself.
2. Ensuring that the capability and capacity of the organisation to undertake the research study or clinical trial, has been met from both a clinical perspective and a research perspective, and that allowing for innovation does not override the requirements for meeting clinical service provision capacity and capability at any time.
3. Ensuring that in circumstances where potential conflicts of interest may exist, particularly where financial or other commercial gain is a possibility, that these have been openly declared and are transparent to the patients and other participants in the study. This is particularly important where there is potential for researchers to receive direct financial reward for the enrolling of patients into a study.

If a patient is harmed or is adversely impacted in any way during a clinical trial or research, there are usually provisions within the research protocol for how such incidents are to be notified to the varying governing bodies oversighting research. Nevertheless, the facility itself must also ensure that standard incident management protocols are in place to support the patient in the event of such an incident. This is particularly important in clinical trials where the patient's adverse incident might be related either directly to the trial itself or to how the clinical care was provided as part of the trial.

The same form and rigour of clinical incident investigation as for clinical care incidents should take place, inclusive of genuine open disclosure and patient-centric incident management. The commitment and goal is to ensure that, where possible, a repeat of such incidents does not occur.

Simply put, research governance, whilst important, is not the only requirement in these circumstances, and healthcare leaders need to ensure that in undertaking research, particularly clinical trials, patients are safe-guarded and managed under the same standard of systems and processes as for receiving direct clinical care.

The collection of activities that govern research at a healthcare organisation is known as a research governance framework.

13.2 Research Governance Frameworks

Health leaders are responsible for developing and enforcing a research governance framework in their organisations. This is to ensure that:

- Any research that is conducted within the organisation is promoted as a valued activity.
- Appropriate training and education of staff in good and ethical research practice is offered and promoted.
- Responsibilities and accountabilities for research activities by individuals and groups are understood, enacted, and maintained.
- Systems and processes that are put in place, are appropriate to the organisation's research environment and sufficiently adaptable to recognise differences in the relative risk of certain types of research (such as interventional research in contrast to observational research).
- All research governance activities are monitored and evaluated, with the framework consequently being modified as appropriate.
- The self-regulation of all contributors to research, upon which the preservation of research integrity depends, is affirmed and can be shown to be practiced.
- The research governance framework is accessible to all relevant parties.
- The rights and reputations of researchers and research participants are respected, and any conflicts of interest are declared and managed.
- The outcomes of research are communicated responsibly.

13.2.1 How to Develop a Research Governance Framework

When designing a research governance framework, it is helpful if health leaders align it to the general stages of a research project lifecycle.

Stage 1 of a research project is usually the research project design (concept).
Stage 2 is the research project authorisation (assessment), which includes consideration of ethical reviews, financial impact, legal and other regulatory requirements, intellectual property rights implications, and risk management.
Stage 3 encompasses the conduct of the research project, where monitoring systems and processes, complaints handling protocols, and reporting requirements are included, and
Stage 4 is often the completion/closure phase of the research project.

Even though it helps to think of these in sequential stages 1–4, the actual implementation of these stages and components is concurrent, and in the development of the framework, it must be taken into account that most of the activities listed will occur in parallel rather than in any prescribed order.

Elements of each stage in the development of an organisation's research governance framework, are described below, to assist healthcare leaders in structuring a practical approach, which they may wish to adopt.

13.2.1.1 Step 1: Initial Assessment of Proposed Research

The initial assessment process that needs to be undertaken by the organisation in undertaking a research project should include:

1. Confirmation of the feasibility and alignment of the research project design to the organisation's and/or clinical department's strategic plans for research.
2. Peer review of scientific, ethical, and practical aspects of the proposed research project.
3. Confirmation that the organisation has the appropriate facilities and other infrastructure or equipment that is required to carry out the research project.
4. Confirmation that the organisation is appropriately staffed to conduct the particular research and to conduct or support any necessary initial and ongoing training.
5. Identification and management of any perceived or actual conflicts of interest.
5. Preparation and review of risk management strategies.
7. Identification of funding sources, including for potential unanticipated costs.
8. Consideration of the suitability of the site for the research project/clinical trial, including how access will be provided to the number of participants required.
9. Establishment of the expectations regarding communication between the Principal Investigator and Research Governance Office, to help streamline processes and reduce duplication.

13.2.1.2 Step 2: Research Project/Clinical Trial Authorisation

This includes developing a process that involves assessing the financial components, ethical aspects, legal and other regulatory requirements, credentialing and supervision of researchers, intellectual property rights implications, and risk management matters. Components that need to be considered include developing specific processes to:

(a) Review the research project/clinical trial budget in preparation for final sign-off by the appropriate finance authority (usually the Director of Finance, Head of Department/Division, and/or delegate).
(b) Complete research grant or other funding processes (where applicable).
(c) Determine fees or cost recovery mechanisms (if applicable) for internal and external service providers.
(d) Identify potential risks of the proposed research activities to the organisation. This includes the selection of appropriate risk management strategies to manage these risks, including consideration of risk transfer or risk sharing (e.g. whether the organisation has appropriate insurance coverage).
(e) Provide relevant indemnities for investigators, where required, based on the organisation's risk profile and chosen management strategy for the research project/clinical trial.

(f) Confirma the roles, responsibilities, and accountabilities for all parties who will be involved in the research project (including investigators, sponsors, and participants).
(g) Affirm the organisation's compliance with relevant guidelines, regulations, legislation, and codes of practice (state and federal).
(h) Complete an accepted standard clinical research agreement (where appropriate).
(i) Comply with notification requirements under the necessary regulatory authority, such as the *Therapeutic Goods Act 1989*, in Australia.
(j) Comply with the requirement to register clinical trials on a publicly accessible clinical trials registry.
(k) Review (and complete) contractual and other legal documentation and confirm that the documentation appropriately reflects the roles, responsibilities, and obligations of each party.
(l) Establish agreements between collaborating institutions as described in the relevant regulation, such as the *Australian Code for the Responsible Conduct of Research, 2017* (including conflicts of interest, defining shared roles and responsibilities, etc.).
(m) Confirm that investigators and support staff have the appropriate qualifications, authorisation/accreditation to practice, and relevant experience.
(n) Confirm arrangements for the supervision and mentoring of any student/junior investigators.
(o) Provide assurance of protection for the organisation's intellectual property.
(p) Negotiate and settle issues about authorship, publication, and potential commercialisation of research.
(q) Comply with the organisation's policy on intellectual property.
(r) Review and provide an opinion on the extent to which the research proposal is ethically acceptable and is compliant with ethical standards and guidelines (termed 'ethical approval').
(s) Determine the need for HREC (Human Research Ethics Committee) review or an appropriate authorised alternate review process (e.g. for low-risk research).
(t) Notify relevant bodies (e.g. in Australia, the Therapeutic Goods Administration), and other institutions participating in the research, of the outcome of ethical review.
(u) Assess each research governance activity, including site-specific assessment and ethical approval, has been satisfactorily completed.
(v) Authorise the research to commence in the organisation and provide the required notifications to the coordinating principal investigator and the clinical executive.

13.2.1.3 Step 3: Research Project/Clinical Trial Conduct

The conduct of the research project requires the framework to define what monitoring systems and processes, complaints handling protocols, and reporting requirements need to be put in place. This includes:

- Monitoring and review of the safety of all research participants and compliance with adverse event reporting requirements.

- Management of research/trial data and storage.
- Management of privacy requirements and maintaining confidentiality of research data.
- Delivery of quality control processes (including supervision of staff and record-keeping).
- Training and/or mentoring of investigators regarding monitoring requirements.
- Monitoring of expenditure and budget.
- Clarification and assignment of responsibility within the organisation for monitoring the conduct/progress of research. Typically, this responsibility is delegated to the Research Governance Office or an equivalent individual or group.
- Demonstration that relevant organisational staff understand and follow the process for information sharing between the organisation, other collaborating institutions, and the ethics committee that conducted the review.
- The coordinating principal investigator has the lead role for communication between the principal investigators at each institution and the ethics committee.
- Compliance with the requirements and timeframes for reporting on project progress.
- Measurement of performance against agreed targets (where appropriate) and modification of processes as needed.
- Compliance with the organisation's process for managing allegations of research misconduct and complaints.
- Incorporation of the principles of natural justice and independence into the management of complaints and allegations.
- Assurance that the complaint process is transparent and communicated to relevant stakeholders and is undertaken in accordance with the requirements set out in the relevant regulation e.g. *Australian Code for the Responsible Conduct of Research.*
- Conduct of self-audit on compliance with good research practice guidelines.
- Compliance with internal and external reporting obligations, including safety reporting and reporting to the ethics committees.
- Provision of training on reporting for investigators and administrators to encourage a culture of oversight and review.

13.2.1.4 Step 4: Research Project/Clinical Trial Completion/Closure

This part of the framework should consider the processes/systems that need to be put in place to ensure:

- Confirmation that project closure is orderly and systematic.
- Completion of an end-of-project checklist.
- Provision of research outcomes to participants (where required).
- Compliance with record storage policies (including future destruction).
- Follow up on intellectual property and commercialisation activities (where applicable).
- Reporting of outcomes to participants, funding bodies, and other stakeholders (where applicable).

Many hospitals and healthcare systems, as part of their value proposition, have a strategic direction to undertake research within their campuses. This commonly includes the involvement of credentialed and practicing clinicians within the healthcare facilities who are undertaking clinical trials. These clinical trials may be initiated by the facility, or more commonly, the facility and the individual clinicians within that facility integrate themselves with an established clinical trial that is being conducted across multiple sites, which usually has external funding. This is particularly the case if a clinical trial has been initiated by a medical device or pharmaceutical company.

Other methods by which research/clinical trials may be undertaken within the organisation include where they have been initiated by a university or via partnerships with universities and other research agencies working collaboratively with the health service facility.

Clinical trials, by their nature, involve patients who are undergoing active treatment for certain conditions or who are being considered for treatment by their treating clinician. Often, these trials require inpatient services to commence or to continue, in terms of either providing the treatment that is under trial, assessing and managing any clinical complications, or other forms of reactions related to the trial. This may also include requirements for undertaking a range of clinical observations within an inpatient unit to monitor the impact of the clinical trial.

Clinical trials and other types of research may also be initiated by a healthcare organisation as part of a clinical service delivery plan, where investment and exploration of innovative and new treatment options, such as the treatment of specific cancers, are part of this overarching plan.

Many organisations that are developing or trialling new treatments will often leverage their connection with the hospital system and individual practitioners to seek access to patients and facilities.

Clinical governance in research is an important element for ensuring the safety of research participants and for ensuring accountability and transparency of practices from the point of view of the researchers themselves. Therefore, it is critical that healthcare organisations undertaking any research within their facilities meet the clinical governance requirements of the facility, in addition to any established broader research governance requirements.

13.3 Case Study 1: Patient Harm in Clinical Trials

A group of oncologists approach your hospital with a proposal to be participants in a clinical trial that has been established for the novel treatment of a complicated form of cancer. This new treatment involves patients who meet specific trial inclusion criteria, being enrolled into a clinical trial. The patients who participate in the trial will be required to be admitted to hospital as inpatients to undertake the treatment. The treatment includes intravenous therapy of a combination of new immunomodulating medications.

There are concerns that the patients may have reactions to the new treatment and therefore they will required to be closely monitored by expert oncology nurses during the time of the infusion and for a period afterwards.

The clinical trial has undergone all research and ethics approvals and has the appropriate authorisations and research governance in place. Your health service is interested to be involved in the clinical trial, as it sees this as keeping with the overall purpose of the organisation and as being aligned with the organisation's strategy. The clinicians involved in the clinical trial are well established at your facility, have a prominent profile, and there is potential for positive reputational impact both for themselves and your organisation, as a result of their involvement in this trial. The trial therefore goes ahead.

Following the first 10 patients treated in the trial, you are notified of a significant clinical incident that involves one of the trial patients, who appear to have suffered a serious setback in their clinical condition, after receiving the experimental medication. Due to this deterioration, for an extensive period of their inpatient admission, they are in the ICU, requiring complex treatment for both the underlying condition as well as the complication of the trial medication.

As the patient was an inpatient, the incident is reported through the usual incident management system, and the investigation by the quality team identifies that there was an error regarding the administration of the drug treatment. It appears that the clinical trial nurse, who is part of the clinical trial program, and who was employed specifically to administer the drug, had in fact incorrectly calculated the dosage and administration rate, and had given the incorrect treatment dose to the patient.

It is apparent that she had been immediately aware of this at the time and had escalated it to her trial coordinator/supervisor, and subsequently, the incident had been reported through the trial governance processes to the Chief Investigator.

Your local investigation determines that the patient had been advised that there had been 'an issue' with the medication which caused the patient's adverse reaction to the medication. However, it is unclear whether this had been noted in the medical record, and to what degree the patient had been advised that there had been an error in the administration dosage.

As this has been escalated to yourself as a senior clinical leader, you initiate your usual incident management processes, including a thorough review of the clinical incident and an assessment of the degree of open disclosure that had been provided to the patient and their family. The clinician involved in the clinical trial is very concerned with respect to the error and wishes to cease their involvement in the trial, as they are concerned that their reputation may be damaged by ongoing participation.

Their colleagues, however, wish for the trial to continue at your facility, as they consider that this error was preventable, and therefore mitigation strategies can be put in place to prevent it from happening again.

Your investigation finds that the clinical trial nurse who gave the incorrect medication is also a staff member of your facility, who works for a clinical trial service under a separate employment contract, and although familiar with your organisation, as they work occasionally in a clinical role, she spends most of her time working in the clinical trials service.

As a result of the investigation, you are satisfied that the requirements for compliance with research governance in this case have been met, and that the clinical trials group have appropriately reported the incident. However, you remain concerned that the incident from a hospital perspective has not been managed correctly or completely, in keeping with your clinical governance processes, and indeed feel that the clinical governance process of the hospital had been superseded by those of the research entity.

You are advised by the clinicians involved in the trial that the research entity and their governance take precedence over that of the hospital and therefore you have "nothing to worry about".

Although you are reassured to some degree, you remain concerned and uneasy that the requirements of your clinical governance processes were not completed. In particular, you note:

1. That the clinical trials staff who undertake the treatments are contracted by an external agency, and whilst there is an agreement between the staff and third-party agency, it is unclear that when present at your facility, whether the clinical trials coordinators understand or are indeed familiar with the clinical policies and procedures in place at your facility. In this case, your investigation shows that the reporting of the clinical incident, escalation of the harm experienced by the patient, and ensuring that the appropriate clinical incident management process had commenced in accordance with your clinical governance process, all appear to have been either ignored, or that those involved had been unfamiliar with the hospital's requirements.
2. It is also unclear how the clinical trials select, orientate, and onboard the clinicians and other staff who are involved in the clinical trial, and in particular, you note that the clinicians are not required to be credentialed to your facility due to the fact that they are employed by the trial group, and are credentialed by that agency.

Your Director of Research advises that they have for some time been planning to introduce a credentialing process for all those undertaking research in the facility regardless of the originating entity. They feel that this will provide a level of assurance with regard to the qualifications, training, and experience of all researchers, and that the researchers are familiar with the policies and procedures of your organisation when conducting research within your facility.

Following this event, you are determined to ensure the same level of scrutiny, investigation, transparency, accountability, and open disclosure, in the event of a clinical trial or any research incident at your facility is equivalent to that of the patient receiving clinical care under normal circumstances.

The legal team at the hospital advises that, in future, contracts with clinical trial entities will be reviewed to ensure that the hospital's requirements for patient management within the facility in the event of a clinical or research incident are managed in the same manner in which the hospital does in normal circumstances. You are assured to learn that this will now be part of the contracting requirements for all similar contracts.

You further act to ensure that the onboarding and orientation of clinical trials staff will be at the same level as those provided for new clinical staff commencing at your health service. Patients will also be advised that although they are enrolled in a clinical trial, their care will be at the same level as if they were routinely admitted for treatment as an inpatient of your facility.

In addition to these issues, you also note that documentation within the clinical record, medication chart, and other systems and processes for good governance in your hospital, had been superseded by the clinical trials requirements. Your review and action ensure that in future, all the documentation that would normally be required by the hospital for an inpatient undergoing treatment, will be completed, and all systems, policies, and procedures will be followed.

There is initial push-back from the trial coordinators and clinicians involved in trials, claiming that this is a form of 'doubling-up' and 'an unnecessary administrative burden'. However, by engaging authentically with those clinicians, and explaining the clinical governance requirements in addition to the research governance requirements, you are able to ensure that an appropriate change management process and improvements to your clinical governance processes are put in place.

Further Reading

Australian Commission on Safety and Quality in Health Care, The National Clinical Trials Governance Framework Pilot and user guide for health service organisations conducting clinical trials. 2022.

National Health and Medical Research Council (NHMRC)/Australian Research Council (ARC)/ Universities Australia Australian Code for the Responsible Conduct of Research, 2007.

National Health and Medical Research Council (NHMRC), Research Governance Handbook: Guidance for the national approach to single ethical review, 2011

Education and Training in Clinical Governance

14

Effective clinical governance demands a commitment to developing and nurturing the skills, knowledge, and attitudes that enable healthcare professionals to deliver safe, effective, patient-centred care. Without a strategic and well-implemented educational framework, even the best-intentioned governance structures will struggle to achieve their objectives.

Education and training that is team based can play an important part in improving patient safety within an organisation. Bringing together clinicians and non-clinicians in scenario, case-based learning ensures that everyone has a better understanding of each other's roles and encourages open communication and dialogue between team members.

Clinicians regularly undertake such team-based training, such as simulation training in the event of a cardiac arrest, as a common example. Simulation-based training provides a safe and controlled environment for practitioners to practice complex procedures and decision-making skills, helping to prevent errors in real-world clinical settings.

However, involving other non-clinical team members in this process ensures that they can align their roles with those of the clinicians involved and have a better understanding of how they can contribute to improve patient outcomes.

Education and training in patient safety play a crucial role in minimising the risk of adverse events. This goes beyond the initial training and certification of healthcare professionals. It requires ongoing, targeted training in areas such as medication safety, infection control, and effective interpersonal communication. Education within this framework should also emphasise the importance of reporting near misses and adverse events without fear of retribution, fostering a learning culture where mistakes are viewed as opportunities for process improvement.

The training programs themselves must be rigorous, evidence-based, and regularly reviewed to ensure that they are aligned with current best practices and evolving patient safety standards. Another crucial element is the training of all staff in recognising and responding to deteriorating patients and ensuring a proactive

© The Author(s), under exclusive license to Springer Nature Singapore Pte Ltd. 2026

L. Prado, S. Chandrasiri, *The Practice of Clinical Governance*,
https://doi.org/10.1007/978-981-19-7896-8_14

approach to patient well-being. Education in clinical governance should move beyond simply attending sessions to encompassing active learning strategies such as reflective practice, case-based discussions, and peer review.

Clinical audits, with their inherent data analysis and interpretation, are significantly more beneficial when staff are trained to interpret findings accurately and utilise them to implement meaningful changes in practice. Training should focus on accessing, interpreting, and applying clinical guidelines and should encourage a culture of questioning current practice and striving for continuous improvement. It should also address the competencies necessary to implement quality improvement initiatives effectively. Specific training in evidence-based medicine is also important, as it allows healthcare practitioners to critically evaluate research and effectively translate findings into improved patient outcomes.

Leaders at all levels of an organisation must understand their responsibilities in promoting a culture of quality and continuous improvement. Leadership training should focus on creating a supportive, learning environment, promoting ethical behaviour and ensuring transparency in decision-making. This includes training in the skills necessary to manage change effectively, facilitate teamwork, and delegate responsibilities appropriately. Clinicians need to be trained in the principles of governance, including the framework for accountability and the consequences of poor practice. Healthcare leaders must also commit resources to ongoing training and demonstrate an active engagement in all aspects of education and continuous development, both for themselves and for their teams.

The organisation needs to ensure that staff members in roles with some component of leadership responsibility, e.g. team leaders, undergo formal education and training in clinical governance, whether that be through academic study or participating in conferences, seminars, and workshops in clinical governance, so that they are well across innovation in this space, and are aware of changes in practice, that can then be introduced into the organisation.

Staff members taking on more encompassing leadership roles will need advanced training in aspects of clinical governance, particularly in the areas of clinical incident management, open disclosure, and complaint handling.

Ensuring leaders are trained to identify potential risks within their specific roles and to implement mitigation strategies effectively is essential. Areas such as digital governance, data protection, and safeguarding vulnerable patients, require specific, ongoing training to ensure compliance with legal and ethical requirements. Education on incident management, including formal reporting and investigation methodologies such as root cause analysis, allows for the identification and correction of system vulnerabilities. Training should focus not just on the technical aspects of risk management but also on the accountabilities leaders hold in promoting a culture of risk awareness and vigilance amongst all staff. This includes specific training on ensuring their teams understand the importance of early escalation of concerns and are aware of how to use the appropriate channels to do so.

Leaders must be able not only to champion clinical governance principles but also to model them in their own practice. Leadership programs should therefore incorporate modules on change management, conflict resolution, and communication strategies. This also extends to developing skills in establishing a 'just culture,' one where staff feel empowered to report errors and concerns without fear of reprisal. Training programs should therefore emphasise the importance of open communication, psychological safety, and learning from mistakes. This involves implementing workshops and training that focus on deconstructing blame culture and promoting a learning environment.

Many clinicians struggle with understanding the complexities of clinical indicators and, in particular, how these indicators can be presented, how they are influenced, how they can be monitored, and how trends can be interpreted and utilised. Therefore, formal education in understanding how to interpret, evaluate, monitor, and utilise clinical indicators is an essential component of clinical governance training. The need for healthcare professionals to maintain their competence and stay abreast of latest advances in medical practice is not just a professional obligation but also a medico-legal imperative. Failure to participate in continuous professional development (CPD) can raise questions about a clinician's competency and knowledge, particularly if their practice differs significantly from current standards. In a negligence case, a lack of CPD can be used to successfully argue that a clinician was not adequately informed or trained to provide the care that was expected of them. This emphasises the importance of having robust systems in place to support CPD and ensuring that records are meticulously maintained. Demonstrable commitment to ongoing learning is crucial for healthcare practitioners and institutions alike.

The practical application of clinical governance, beyond the theoretical frameworks, forms the bedrock of impactful clinical governance training.

This necessitates that staff are trained on specific tools and techniques applicable to daily practice. For example, staff involved in clinical incident reporting need to be trained on specific methodologies such as root cause analysis (RCA), and the '5 Whys' technique or fishbone diagrams. This training must extend beyond basic instruction and facilitate the development of competence in using these tools effectively and consistently. Similarly, training on audit methodology should enable professionals to not just perform audits but also to interpret findings critically, develop realistic action plans, and monitor their effectiveness. This means moving away from merely completing audit cycles and towards understanding how audits can catalyse tangible service improvements. This practical application must also encompass the use of data analytics to identify areas for improvement and to track progress against identified goals. Data literacy, therefore, becomes a crucial component of any relevant training.

The field of clinical governance is constantly evolving, necessitating continuous development of skills and knowledge. Health leaders must remain abreast of emerging trends and best practices through advanced professional development programs. This includes training on new technologies (e.g., AI in healthcare, telehealth), implementation of evidence-based guidelines, and understanding evolving patient safety standards. Further, medical administrators need to be trained on the intricacies of multi-professional working and collaboration to ensure a holistic approach to clinical governance. This can involve interprofessional simulation exercises designed to mimic real-world healthcare scenarios, where different professionals can work together to identify and mitigate potential risks. This kind of training promotes collaborative practice and ensures a unified approach to standards of care across all service areas. This training should, in fact, adapt to diverse contexts and reflect the unique challenges faced by specific healthcare settings.

The training needs of a large teaching hospital will differ significantly from those of a community-based clinic. Hence, customised programmes that reflect local needs and resources are crucial. Health leaders should also be versed in the use of effective needs analysis methodologies to allow for tailored training programs. This requires a deep understanding of the organisational structure and processes, as well as the clinical expertise of those being trained. This ensures training is relevant, engaging, and ultimately effective in improving clinical outcomes. Finally, the evaluation of training programs must move beyond simple feedback forms and adopt more rigorous methods. Measuring the impact of the education on actual change in clinical practice is essential. This can involve monitoring specific quality indicators, conducting pre- and post-training audits, and assessing changes in staff attitudes and behaviours.

The focus should be on demonstrating a tangible return on investment in clinical governance training, in terms of measurable improvements in care quality and patient outcomes. This continuous evaluation cycle is crucial, ensuring improvements are made to training programs based on data and feedback. Education and training in clinical governance is not a one-time event but an ongoing journey of continuous improvement. For healthcare leaders in the field, this necessitates embracing a commitment to continuous learning and leading the charge in developing and implementing rigorous, evidence-based programs. These programs must not only impart knowledge, but also embed practical skills and promote leadership qualities that are conducive to a culture of safety, transparency, and continuous improvement, ultimately ensuring the highest standards of care for all patients. Moving beyond the theoretical framework and into practical implementation and critical evaluation is key to realising the true potential of clinical governance. This demands a proactive and strategic approach that sees training and education in clinical governance as an investment in continuous improvement and, ultimately, better patient care.

14.1 Communication in Safety and Quality

To engage all levels across all professional groups, including non-clinicians, in safety and quality, it is important to ensure that there is a regular form of communication with staff. Traditionally, many organisations use a form of 'newsletter' to pass on new information or highlight a particular topic. Other approaches such as posters, flyers, screen savers and dedicated web-pages, and similar 'advertising' are widely used in hospitals. However, these are 'one-dimensional' and do not allow for discussion, questions, and true engagement.

Many organisations will include safety and quality topics in orientation, mandatory training within educational forums (such as open disclosure), whilst some will have safety weeks/months with the focus often rotating through a number of themes such as falls, medication safety etc.

Few organisations measure the effectiveness of their communication and their actual impact on practice and outcomes. Often a program of education on a particular clinical governance topic will follow an investigations of a clinical incident, leading to new policies, procedures, forms etc. 'Formal education' commonly therefore forms a part of the formal recommendations as an outcome of such an investigation.

All this leads to a flurry of activity, bombarding staff with messages, and often the 'changes' hoped for are either not long lasting and rarely measured, or if indeed measured, feedback linking the training to change is often not provided.

Effective training, communication, engagement, and participation of staff in clinical governance is essential. Such programs should be assessed for effectiveness and practical impact, for example, as part of a survey of the culture of safety and quality across the organisation, with specific questions being included on education and communication.

14.2 Orientation and On-Boarding

Organisations can set the tone of the importance of clinical governance by incorporating this topic in their orientation and on-boarding programs for new staff members. Including specific wording around the commitment to safety and quality within position descriptions, regardless of the role, and highlighting this alignment to the organisation's values, purpose, and vision, enables the new recruit to understand that their role is critically linked to ensuring safety and quality of care provided to patients. Those in leadership roles should be clear that safety and quality is a part of their responsibilities, as well as the importance of leaders setting the right tone, with clear accountabilities and measurable KPIs.

Orientation and on-boarding programs should include a clear commitment to safety and quality, and how all staff are involved and how staff will be engaged in ensuring this. Highlighting how staff can raise concerns and escalate to the appropriate leaders, is an important part of the orientation.

Senior leaders and executives should involve themselves in the orientation process, as messaging on this topic from this level of leadership sends a strong and clear statement to new staff. Orientation is also an ideal and indeed critical time to highlight key safety and quality policies and procedures, such as hand hygiene, whilst also undertaking required mandatory training in safety and quality, such as, for example, basic life support and medication prescribing. It is important that sufficient time is given to orientation and on-boarding to allow for staff to absorb information. The value and importance of orientation and on-boarding process cannot be overstated, and therefore the effectiveness of orientation should be continuously evaluated and appropriate improvements made to its structure, content and delivery.

14.3 Mandatory Training

Organisations use mandatory training to reinforce important educational messages; therefore, it is common that mandatory training include safety and quality topics. Mandatory training is usually completed at least on a yearly basis, and therefore it is important that topics are reviewed each year, with the content being updated. Including safety and quality topics in mandatory training will highlight their importance; however, mandatory training is often considered bothersome by staff, and therefore it is critical to ensure that topics remain relevant and of interest to them. This can be achieved by the use of case studies and patient stories which resonate with staff and help provide context and relevance to their training.

14.4 Formal Education

Organisations should ensure that a robust program of education on clinical governance topics is made available as part of education offerings, and where necessary, there are opportunities provided for professional development of staff on clinical governance, including external courses and programs. Incorporating clinical governance topics in leadership training programs is of significant importance to embed safety and quality across the organisation. If internal programs are not available, then external agencies should be utilised. Communication skills training is an important component of such educational programmes. This is particularly the case for dealing with difficult conversations such as managing disruptive behaviour and undertaking open disclosure processes following clinical incidents. Where possible, educational programs should include team-based learning and case studies. Involving patients and consumers in such training is also beneficial.

Whilst formal programs are important, on-the-job training, where every possible clinical scenario, clinical review, and incident is used as an opportunities to teach and learn, is vital. This can assist with reinforcing previous learnings and giving context for the practical adaptation of theoretical concepts. Such training can greatly assist preparing staff for how to manage when faced with practical realities, such as being able to manage difficult interactions.

Further Reading

Pearce, Paddy, and McSherry, Robert. Clinical Governance: A Guide to Implementation for Healthcare Professionals. Germany, Wiley, 2011.

Clinical Governance in Artificial Intelligence

15

Artificial Intelligence (AI) refers to the simulation of human intelligence processes by machines, particularly computer systems. It involves the development of algorithms and technologies that enable computers to perform tasks that typically require human intelligence. AI systems can learn from data, adapt to new information, and make decisions or predictions based on that data. The promise of AI is the development of machines that can mimic cognitive functions like learning, reasoning, problem-solving, perception, and language understanding.

Three main components and approaches commonly being utilised by AI in healthcare include combinations of machine learning, deep learning, and natural language processing. These pose significant safety and quality challenges for healthcare organisations.

Machine Learning (ML) Machine learning focuses on developing algorithms that allow computers to learn patterns from data and extrapolate these to make predictions of further patterns. These algorithms improve their performance over time as they are exposed to more data. In healthcare, the most common application of traditional machine learning is in the area of 'precision medicine'—predicting which treatment protocols are likely to succeed for a patient based on various patient attributes and the treatment context.

Deep Learning Deep learning is a subfield of machine learning that processes and analyses complex data, particularly images and text, which allows for the detection and diagnosis of medical conditions/pathologies such as in medical imaging eg CT and MRI scans. Incorporating AI into medical imaging allows the function of deep learning to be used, for example, in the detection of melanomas and brain tumours that may not be easily perceived by the human eye.

© The Author(s), under exclusive license to Springer Nature Singapore Pte Ltd. 2026

L. Prado, S. Chandrasiri, *The Practice of Clinical Governance*,
https://doi.org/10.1007/978-981-19-7896-8_15

Natural Language Processing (NLP) NLP involves enabling computers to understand, interpret, and generate human language, which can be used in healthcare for dictating documentation and translating speech-to-text. A broader use of NLP includes the ability to analyse electronic health records, for example, to improve the accuracy of identifying unexpected hospital readmissions, predicting length of stay, and forecasting inpatient mortality.

The use of AI in healthcare is rapidly evolving. Some of these areas and real-life utilisation examples include:

Predictive Analytics Forecasting seasonal spikes in flu cases, enabling hospitals to proactively allocate beds and staffing, thus minimising emergency room overcrowding and improving patient flow.

Monitoring and Alerts Monitoring of patients in critical care settings and using clinical data in real-time, flagging anomalies and potential complications that may require immediate action.

Access and Flow Optimisation Scrutinising patient flow and staffing patterns to predict optimal staffing levels for specific periods, allowing hospitals to avoid understaffing or overstaffing and thereby optimising resource allocation.

Adverse Event Prevention Analysing data on patient outcomes, adverse events, and a hospital's adherence to clinical guidelines, to identify causal associations and to pinpoint areas where adjustments and improvements are needed.

Experience-Driven Personalised Care Scanning diverse datasets, including genomics, lifestyle factors, past treatment responses and patient experience outcomes, to identify the most effective treatment plan for individual patients.

As the efficacy and use of artificial intelligence (AI) in improving aspects of healthcare delivery becomes more and more evident, AI will increasingly become incorporated into routine clinical care. Concerns about the ethical and regulatory aspects of the application of AI in healthcare is therefore increasingly coming to the forefront.

15.1 Ethical Challenges

There are three key ethical challenges that healthcare leaders will need to navigate in ensuring that AI applications are incorporated into routine clinical care under appropriate clinical governance. These include AI bias, data privacy, and maintaining the professional trust between patients and clinicians. All these pose risks and opportunities from a clinical safety and quality perspective.

AI bias arises when the data used for analysis or processing are not representative of the target population, or when inadequate or incomplete data is used in the building of AI models. Under-representative data can often occur in situations where, for example, societal discrimination (leading to poor access to healthcare), and relatively small sample sizes (such as with minority groups), have been used. Such biased algorithms may then lead to an underestimation or overestimation of risks in certain patient populations. Reducing AI bias will therefore be necessary for promoting both better and more equitable health outcomes, and to avoid unexpected or unintended patient harm.

Data privacy is key to ensuring the maintenance of patient confidentiality and to obtaining genuine informed consent from patients, both for health interventions and for the usage of their personal health information. Healthcare systems that use AI should therefore be protected from privacy breaches, and allow for mechanisms where patients are able to provide explicit consent for their personal data to be used for any specific purpose.

Patient and clinician trust involves transparency in the clinical decision-making process and in the shared conversation between clinicians and patients when explaining and discussing diagnostic and treatment processes. The nature of AI algorithms, especially deep learning algorithms, is such that they continuously fine-tune their parameters and continue to evolve the rules of learning. This can lead to opaque decision-making processes. If clinicians do not understand the inner workings of AI models, they may be unable to understand or explain the reasoning behind the diagnostic and medical treatment processes that are determined by AI for their patients. Additionally, an overreliance on AI models may reduce or eliminate the compassionate contact and empathic conversation between clinicians and patients, which is crucial for good patient care and enabling patient autonomy.

15.2 Regulatory Challenges

Given the ability of AI used in healthcare to auto-learn from its use in the real world, in order to continuously improve its performance and update its decision-making algorithms over time, developing a set policies and guidelines that regulate its use, becomes quickly redundant. Regulatory standards that are currently available for assessing the safety and impact of AI algorithms are largely still unverified, and not formalised. This presents a significant clinical governance challenge for healthcare leaders in relation to mitigating any unsafe practices of AI use in their healthcare services.

The issue of liability as to who is responsible in the event of any adverse clinical outcomes arising from errors or failures in the use of AI-enabled tools, is an additional concern.

In the absence of clear and fit-for-purpose regulatory and accreditation systems and guidelines, rapid progress in the development, deployment, and use of AI models in healthcare presents several clinical governance concerns and challenges for health leaders.

15.3 Developing a Clinical Governance Framework for AI Adoption

Given the nascent stages of regulation, standards, and guidelines to assist healthcare leaders validate, introduce, monitor, and evaluate any AI-enabled components that are incorporated into clinical practice, adherence to the clinical governance principles, for example, as set out in the National Model Clinical Governance Framework for Australia, is suggested.

As outlined in earlier chapters, it is important to recognise the positioning and overlap of clinical governance with financial, risk, and other corporate governance imperatives. The clinical governance system of a health service or organisation can be conceptualised as a system within a system, where clinical governance is a system that intersects with financial governance, risk governance, and the overall corporate governance system.

In considering the development of appropriate governance systems for enabling and supporting the use of AI in healthcare, financial and risk evaluations of the specific form/aspect of AI that is being used should also be evaluated.

This is primarily due to the fact that decisions about these aspects of corporate governance can have a direct effect on the safety and quality of care and vice versa, as has been outlined in earlier chapters.

Financial governance considerations of AI would include consideration of such attributes as upfront capital/software costs and maintenance costs specific to the AI component (including installation, training, and internal resourcing), in addition to any costs involved in ensuring inter-operability within existing IT systems and/or retirement of legacy systems. This should also take into consideration resourcing costs from an expertise perspective, as well as costs that are involved in ensuring that a robust cybersecurity framework and system is in place prior to the introduction of any new AI.

Evaluation should include ROI (return on investment), that assesses not only any financial benefits gained as a result of investment in AI, but also the equivalent monetary value of any improved processes, any enhanced reputational impacts for the organisation, any benefits gained by improved user experience, and any potential cost reductions as a result of process/equipment/system replacements. This will also lead to a better understanding of the financial 'cost' of safety and quality impact of AI.

Legal and Risk governance considerations of AI would include ensuring adherence to existing regulations and standards governing the use of AI in healthcare. This is in addition to ensuring that systems and processes that are capable of keeping pace with the rapid advancement of regulations and the introduction of standards related to AI, are also put in place.

Identifying and creating management strategies, as well as contingency plans, to address the risks in each of these areas, is critical:

Data Security Risks Mechanisms to protect patients' personal information and comply with local and national data protection laws and regulations.

Infrastructure Security Risks Mechanisms to identify and manage any vulnerabilities when integrating with or incorporating into existing IT infrastructure.

Legal Risks Including definitions of data ownership, responsibilities for clinical decision-making using AI software or AI guidance, and overall medico-legal and indemnity coverage for adverse events arising as a result of using AI guidance or involvement in clinical decision-making processes.

Regulatory Risks This is particularly challenging, given the need to ensure ongoing compliance with rapidly changing regulatory requirements in the AI space.

Reputational Risks Strategies developed to proactively communicate the benefits of adopting AI to both internal and external stakeholders of the healthcare organisation are crucial in managing any potential damage to the organisation's reputation and standing in the community.

15.4 Clinical Governance Considerations

15.4.1 Governance, Leadership, and Culture

In the development and application of clinical governance systems for incorporating AI in healthcare, all stakeholders, from health boards, executive teams, clinicians, staff, as well as consumers, need to be authentically engaged. This further extends to community and primary care sectors, when the AI adoptiion may have an impact across these external networks. This includes the individual and collective responsibilities for ensuring clinical governance of AI use, by primary care providers, allied health providers, community providers, aged care facilities, and other healthcare providers, depending on the type of linkages that exist already with the health service where the AI is being introduced.

15.4.2 Patient Safety and Quality Improvement Systems

Appropriate mechanisms for the validation of AI systems are critical in ensuring that their functionality, which impacts patient care, is safe, effective, and patient-centred. Validation helps to ensure that the system will function as intended and that there are processes in place to identify any potential issues (such as malfunctions) that could result in an adverse outcome to the patient. Should an issue arise, these should able to be formally recorded and managed, and any improvements should be able to be implemented and tracked. The incident management system needs to incorporate the recording and management of incidents particularly where there may be significant AI involvement as a separate functionality. Policies, procedures, and clinical care guidelines for governing these functions in relation to AI, including escalation of concerns, open disclosure, feedback, and complaints management, will need to be developed.

The role of the government health regulatory bodies such as the Food and Drug Administration (FDA) in the United States and the Therapeutic Goods Administration (TGA) in Australia, in the validation of AI-augmented new technologies or devices prior to their introduction into healthcare settings, will need to be defined, including provisions for mutual recognition of any similar overseas regulatory approvals.

Establishment of a governance system for the safe introduction of AI-augmented software or modification of existing new technology governance systems within health services themselves, will also be required, including the incorporation of any third-party/other expertise from a resourcing perspective, to ensure an adequate, relevant, and robust assessment and evaluation process is in place.

Existing clinical governance and committee reporting structures where AI related incidents are reported, reviewed, and evaluated would need to consider incorporating relevant IT and/or AI/digital health expertise to review the aspects of escalated concerns that may relate specificaly to AI governance. Whether this linkage extends to external and proprietary owners of the AI software via third-party agreements (or service level agreements), would also need consideration, depending on the specific type and function of AI that is being adopted.

Obtaining and documenting informed consent from patients, detailing the extent and nature of any AI augmentation in their clinical care, will require specific consideration, with options for patients to opt out of AI-augmented care models should they wish to do so at any time, being made available.

Similarly, a conscientious objection process permitting abstaining from the use of any AI-augmented clinical care component may need to be considered for clinicians who may object to the use of AI as part of upholding clinician autonomy in providing clinical care. The impact of this would, of course, vary depending on the nature, extent, and functionality of the AI-augmented clinical care component that is in question.

15.4.3 Clinical Performance and Effectiveness

The health workforce that will be utilising the functionality afforded by the particular AI guidance, will need to be appropriately credentialed and trained in its use. Delineation of scopes of clinical practice will require modifications to ensure any clinical decision-making or procedural techniques that are performed using AI guidance and input, are specifically identified and recorded as part of the clinician's scope of practice.

Seeking additional evidence of qualifications or advanced training in using and/or providing supervision, on a particular aspect of AI in providing clinical care, may need to be defined. Speciality colleges may have a role in determining specific training requirements for medical practitioners based on the particular AI functionality that is being adopted within specialities and specific medical diagnostics or surgical procedures in question.

Health service credentialing committees (and equivalent structures) will need to consider IT/AI technicians and clinicians as part of credentialing committee memberships. The need to ensure the safe maintenance of AI systems as well as corresponding cybersecurity measures may require the expansion or repurposing of IT/digital health personnel across healthcare teams and across various committee structures.

Medical practitioners' and health services' medico-legal liabilities and indemnity cover for the use of AI-guided clinical care will require modification from both a health service insurance perspective as well as an individual practitioner indemnity insurance perspective.

Internal and external benchmarking of clinical outcomes arising from AI-enhanced clinical care, comparison, and monitoring trends of relevant KPIs (key performance indicators), and establishing appropriate case conferences, multidisciplinary meetings, and clinical audits, for evaluating the ongoing use of AI-enabled clinical care, are further aspects that need to be considered in ensuring safe clinical performance within a robust clinical governance framework.

15.4.4 Safety and Quality Considerations

The maturity and responsiveness of the IT and cybersecurity infrastructure of health services providing AI-augmented clinical services, will assist in delineating the clinical capability frameworks of the services that can be safely provided at a particular health service site. This would include the establishment of backup systems should the AI-enabled clinical care delivery system fail or malfunction at any point, with safe business continuity plans and critical equipment failure response processes established.

Pre-emptive and routine checks for identifying software glitches, electronic failures, and potential bias in AI decision-making systems will need to be developed, along side the processes established for regular monitoring and updating.

There are a number of key areas that could lead to potential adverse clinical incidents that relate to the use of AI in healthcare systems. In ensuring a robust clinical governance framework to address these, healthcare leaders should specifically consider the following:

1. *Data bias* as mentioned above, is a potential major cause of adverse events, as AI algorithms are reliant on limited historical data. If this data contains underlying socioeconomic or other biases, the AI system will learn and perpetuate these biases. The consequence of such bias is significant for potential misdiagnosis or creating unequal access to effective treatments for certain patient populations. Such bias may then result in a direct negative impact on all patient outcomes.
2. *Errors in data entry, implementation of algorithms, and system maintenance* are important potential risks to patient safety from an AI system. Input errors, such as inaccurate patient demographic and clinical data, can cause significant clinical impact through the erroneous conclusions that may be reached as a result. Inaccurate labelling of training data can also introduce bias and reduce algorithm

accuracy. Without a proper system for periodic review and maintenance of AI systems, the reliability of AI tools may reduce, increasing the risk of adverse incidents.

3. *User error and insufficient clinician training* are key risks. Clinicians must be adequately trained on how to interpret and use the outputs of AI systems. Otherwise, they may incorrectly apply the outcomes from the AI system, leading to adverse events.
4. *Over-reliance on AI* from the phenomenon of automation bias can arise where clinicians may accept and follow the recommendations of an AI tool without employing critical thinking skills, even when those recommendations would be considered inappropriate based on their clinical expertise and understanding of the specifics in a case. AI systems should be designed to support clinician decision-making and should not be seen as a replacement for clinician judgement and experience. Therefore, adequate on-going training is needed.
5. A significant concern revolves around the '*black box*' nature of many AI algorithms. These data models often lack transparency in how their decision-making processes are undertaken. This therefore may lead the clinician to not understand why a certain output has been determined by the AI system, which may adversely impact the care provided. On the other hand, if a clinician is not aware of this potential risk, they may not question any decisions made by the AI system, and this itself may lead to an adverse clinical outcome.

15.4.5 Partnering with Consumers

New systems and processes, or modifications to existing systems and processes that are used in supporting patients, carers, and families in navigating their healthcare journeys, will need to be developed. This will include partnering with patients and consumers in AI health literacy, developing specific patient information, and providing transparency and explanations of the algorithms used by a particular AI-enhanced decision-making tool. This is essential to ensure that patients retain their involvement and input in directing their own care.

Training medical practitioners and clinicians in talking to patients and families about the role that AI may play in their particular health journeys will be crucial, as well as training and relevant measures being implemented to ensure that the clinician continues to retain primary responsibility for all clinical decision-making.

Health service leaders may further wish to involve patients and consumers from the outset, in determining their organisation's readiness and planning for adopting AI-enabled devices or software, by offering opportunities to participate in relevant committees, seeking active feedback, and/or via focus or consumer advisory groups.

Healthcare organisations must invest in training clinicians on the appropriate use of AI tools, including how to interpret and critique AI recommendations, and how to recognise when an AI system might be making an error. Clear protocols for human oversight of AI-driven care and protocols for managing situations when AI systems are unavailable or malfunction, are essential.

Finally, continuous auditing mechanisms and feedback loops that enable AI systems to learn from errors and improve over time, are also critical for achieving the intended benefits of AI without compromising patient safety. In conclusion, the implementation of AI in healthcare undoubtedly has the potential to provide better, more efficient, and more personalised care to patients. Nevertheless, proactively anticipating and addressing the potential for adverse incidents, is crucial in realising this potential safely and responsibly.

Further Reading

Sandeep Reddy, Sonia Allan, Simon Coghlan, and Paul Cooper. A governance model for the application of AI in health care. J Am Med Inform Assoc. 2020 Mar; 27(3): 491–497

Char DS, Shah NH, Magnus D. Implementing machine learning in healthcare-addressing ethical challenges. *N Engl J Med* 2018; 378 (11): 981–3.

Liao F, Adelaine S, Afshar M and Patterson BW (2022) Governance of Clinical AI applications to facilitate safe and equitable deployment in a large health system: Key elements and early successes.

https://healthitanalytics.com/features/what-is-deep-learning-and-how-will-it-change-healthcare

Australian Commission on Safety and Quality in Health Care. National Model Clinical Governance Framework. Sydney: ACSQHC; 2017.

Cunha Renato. AI Governance for Healthcare: A Comprehensive Framework. Linkedin Article. April 17, 2023.

16 Clinical Governance in Non-hospital and Other Healthcare Settings

Increasingly complex healthcare is being delivered 'outside of the hospital's walls'. Examples include chemotherapy and antibiotic treatments being provided in the patient's home or at a community based ambulatory care center. Since the Covid pandemic there has been a significant increase in the provision of 'out of hospital' services such as 'virtual wards', 'virtual' emergency departments, and 'hospital in the home'. There has also been a rapid rise in clinical consultations via telehealth, including post discharge follow ups. Primary care practices and community care centers have also seen an increase in the complexity of care that they are providing, especially with the challenges of gaining admission of patients to hospital, and the additional responsibility for complex care being provided in the community. Increasingly, there are greater community, government, and professional expectations that evidence of practical implementation of high standards of safety and quality, occurs in all health care settings. Therefore, ensuring that an effective clinical governance framework, including robust processes for ensuring accountability for clinical governance, is in place for 'out of hospital settings' is important.

There are many 'out of hospitals' settings. These include primary care, ambulatory care, out-patients, community services, medical specialist practices, and aged care facilities. As mentioned above, the patient's own 'home' is now increasingly the location of where care is provided. For the purpose of this chapter, the focus will be on just two of these settings: 'Primary Care' and 'Virtual Care', noting that each of the 'settings' listed above have unique requirements and challenges. Nevertheless, considering these two 'settings' allows for an understanding of the 'general' requirements for clinical governance in *non-hospital* settings, and also shines a light on some of the complexities faced by leaders in such settings. In general, and in part due to the rapid establishment of these programs, these 'out-of-hospital' healthcare settings may be particularly challenged with implementing

© The Author(s), under exclusive license to Springer Nature Singapore Pte Ltd. 2026
L. Prado, S. Chandrasiri, *The Practice of Clinical Governance*,
https://doi.org/10.1007/978-981-19-7896-8_16

a clinical governance framework and with ensuring that it is effectively monitored. These challenges can include:

1. Insufficient understanding, knowledge, and training in clinical governance.
2. Varying levels of capabilities of leaders and staff and the paucity of resources available to them.
3. Navigating and managing the range of complex governance and reporting structures that often involve multiple regulatory authorities, accreditation bodies, licensing agencies, and other various stakeholders.

Given the increasing expectations for clinical governance in these 'out of hospital' settings, the following general principles are useful in the practical implementation of clinical governance systems:

1. Clear clinical governance responsibilities are articulated throughout the organisation.
   (a) Clinical governance accountabilities, roles, and responsibilities are clear at the 'governing board' level, through executive, management and throughout the organisation.
   (b) Relevant key clinical outcome indicators are monitored, reviewed, and actioned at all levels.
   (c) Appropriate resources in terms of staff and support systems are made available and put in place.
   (d) Each member of staff is aware of and accountable for their role in clinical governance.
2. External regulatory standards are monitored and reviewed.
   (a) Robust processes are in place for monitoring changes with regulatory requirements as relevant to the type of healthcare setting, e.g. aged care facility accreditation.
   (b) Responsibility for ensuring the compliance requirements are clear and are reviewed by the accountable level of governance within the organisation e.g. the Board.
3. Culture of safety and quality is evident throughout the organisation.
   (a) All staff are able to escalate concerns regarding safety and quality, are clear on how to undertake this, and that feedback and actions are implemented and closed off.
   (b) Staff are regularly surveyed in terms of their thoughts on the organisational culture.
   (c) Staff are actively involved in promoting, and are authentically consulted on improvements in safety and quality.
4. Consumers are actively engaged and participate in safety and quality.

   (a) A robust process is in place for the consumers receiving the healthcare services to complain, comment, and provide feedback on safety and quality.
   (b) Consumers are represented on the appropriate governance structures and committees relating to safety and quality.
   (c) Consumers are actively involved in the review of performance, incident management, and improvement activities.

5. Risk management, incident investigation and analysis systems and processes are robust.

   (a) The organisation's risk framework informs and is aligned to the clinical governance framework, and that incident management processes are robust and meets current best practice.

General Structure and Framework
Regardless of the out of hospital healthcare setting, the following standard framework is recommended when structuring a clinical governance system, including ensuring a minimum level of consumer participation:

1. Committee structure
   Highest governance entity e.g. Board.

   - Relevant subcommittee for safety and quality/clinical governance.
   - Executive management committee.
   - Subcommittee for safety and quality/clinical governance,
   - Consumer experience and engagement committee.
   - Incident/complaints management committee.

2. Key roles

   - CEO/senior Executive.
   - Executive/director level responsible for clinical governance.
   - Manager of healthcare delivery (responsible for outcomes and experience, incidents and complaints, compliance, policies/procedures/audits).
   - Manager of safety and quality (or combined with above depending on organisation size).

3. Key policies and procedures

   - Overarching clinical governance framework.
   - Risk management framework and incident management and investigation framework.
   - Accreditation and standards compliance framework.
   - Consumer engagement and participation framework.
   - Complaints feedback process.
   - Safety and quality procedures specific to the organisation.

16.1 Primary Care Settings

Primary care facilities are generally considered fundamental providers of general care in the community. These can vary from solo practices to large group practices, providing multidisciplinary care with extensive additional services, such as radiology, and undertaking increasingly significant procedures, such as iron infusions.

In some countries, such as Australia, primary care facilities undergo accreditation processes, usually involving a site visit, to review their clinical governance framework and its practical application. A positive outcome may result in financial incentive benefits from government agencies and other funders, in terms of additional payments or access to additional programs.

For those who are responsible for primary care services, including solo practitioners, there is a need to ensure robust clinical governance is in place, to provide for compliance with relevant regulatory requirements and also from a litigation, medico-legal perspective. Despite the challenges of primary care, including the risk of 'isolation' that be an issue for solo and small group practices, an appropriate clinical governance framework can be formulated and put in place.

16.2 Key Clinical Governance Principles

It is important to ensure that there is a clearly designated lead for clinical governance. This may be the most senior clinician or healthcare provider within the setting. This role should undergo at least basic training in clinical governance and be familiar with the key components of clinical governance as outlined in this book. Their role includes:

1. Ensuring regular team meetings are held to discuss healthcare provided and how this can be improved. Exploring opportunities to undertake benchmarking and collaboration with similar-sized organisations as needed.
2. Identifying risks, particularly clinical risk, in relation to the services provided. Examining the risks for any new services being considered. Ensuring that adequate training is provided for those providing care and that they are supported with appropriate resources, such as emergency equipment.
3. Researching best practices undertaken in the type of healthcare being provided and benchmarking current practices. Using the published 'learnings' and available evidence to review and improve practice.
4. Selecting important, manageable performance indicators that will provide assurance of how clinical governance framework is functioning.
5. Instigating a process for the review of incidents, complaints, and other issues for investigation and improvement.

Aged-care facilities and similar residential services must ensure that:

- Consumer, client, and patient engagement and how services are provided are transparent, and that there is evidence of this in practice.

- Family, friends, caregivers, and next-of-kin have access to healthcare providers to raise their concerns, provide feedback, suggest improvements, and are engaged in monitoring how services are provided.
- Clear pathways for escalation of deterioration in clinical states are in place, and processes for transfer to higher levels of care are robust.
- Client and patient expectations regarding their healthcare are well known to care teams and articulated to ensure all are aware of and respond appropriately.
- A clear framework is in place to meet the requirements of audit and compliance with aged care sector requirements.
- Ongoing training, including simulation training for caregivers, is in place, e.g. when a new policy or procedure is introduced.
- Clear communication and collaboration processes with external healthcare providers, including primary care, allied health, and pharmacy, are in place to avoid miscommunication and to maximise the standard of care provided.

16.3 Case Study 1: New Service Provision in Primary Care

A primary care family practice wishes to introduce iron infusions to provide to their patients who meet clinical criteria for iron deficiency, as access to such treatment currently depends on the public hospital which is experiencing significant wait time for an appointment. According to the Group Practices' clinical governance framework, the following steps and actions are undertaken:

- The clinical director of the group takes the lead with the introduction of the service.
- The Group's clinicians, doctors, nurses, and administration staff discuss the proposal at their regular patient safety improvement meeting.
- An agreed position that the service should be introduced if all clinical governance facilities are in place is reached.
- An agreed set of clinical criteria is determined for current best practice and shared for discussion and ongoing review.
- The practice nurse is tasked with identifying best practices in iron infusions at both hospital and primary care sites, including policies and procedures, for review and adaptation by the practice.
- Clinical risks of the treatment, such as 'staining' and 'anaphylaxis' during infusion, are identified, and the appropriate mitigation strategies such as policies, training, and supervision requirements are defined.
- Adequate and appropriate resources and equipment to insert cannulas and to perform resuscitation if needed, are considered.
- Appropriate consent, patient information, and the process for explaining risks and benefits are developed.
- Processes for appropriate administrative issues such as appointment scheduling and cost management are developed.

- Agreed clinical outcomes to be monitored, such as levels of ferritin pre- and post-treatment, and arrangements for follow-up care are determined.
- A process for reviewing clinical incidents as they occur and for reviewing the service at agreed intervals is agreed upon and documented.
- Agreed clinical pathways of care and workflows, e.g. cannula size, location, and infusion rates, are developed.

This case study outlines an example of safely introducing a new clinical service to a non-hospital setting within an appropriate clinical governance framework that ensures quality of care, in a safe and patient-centric environment.

Key Lessons
The principles of clinical governance apply to all healthcare settings.

1. By utilising these principles in a proactive manner, the health leaders of primary care services can assure safe, quality care, improvement in care, prevention of adverse incidents, and meeting external regulatory standards and requirements.
2. Involving a multidisciplinary team of clinicians and administrative staff, led by a dedicated person who is responsible and accountable for clinical governance, provides for the best governance structure.
3. Using a patient-centric approach, reviewing risk, benchmarking, and ensuring adequate training and resources ensures safe practice.

16.4 Case Study 2: Infection Outbreak in an Aged Care Service

A large residential care facility experiences an outbreak of COVID-19 infections in both staff and residents, resulting in close to 100 persons returning a positive test over a matter of days. As a consequence, the jurisdictional head of healthcare orders that infected staff and all close contacts be isolated at home, leading to the entire clinical workforce being removed from duty. Given the emergency response, an external agency is tasked with bringing staff into the facility to care for the residents in the meantime.

As the outbreak spreads amongst the residents, a number succumbs to the infection, and the number of deaths increases. Because of the outbreak and resulting impact on residents, the jurisdiction triggers an 'evacuation' plan to move residents into available private hospital beds. The process of evacuation involves state and national health department officials, local facility managers (although they worked for the agency), senior clinicians from the agency and ambulance services. Over the next 48 hours, residents are evacuated according to clinical criteria to hospitals.

Deaths of residents within days of evacuation occurres. An investigation following this event uncovers a number of clinical governance failures. These include:

1. The primary care providers that usually cared for the residents were not involved in the process of outbreak management or evacuation.
2. There was a lack of clinical care plans with respect to 'end of life' care for individual residents, which therefore left the receiving hospitals' clinicians 'in the dark' in relation to the residents' wishes. This was exacerbated with regard to the lack of interaction with the primary care providers.
3. Families and next of kin were not engaged with regards to the residents' evacuation and care plans. The impact of COVID-related visiting restrictions, resulted in an ongoing disconnect between families and clinicians caring for the residents.
4. Agency staff were not familiar with the residents and their families. Consequently, the policies and procedures for how residents' identifications were checked, how medications were managed, how healthcare services were provided, infection prevention protocols, clinical escalation processes, and general safety and quality processes were undertaken were essentially unknown and had to be developed 'on the run'. This resulted in significant delays in treatment, and confusion with regards to chronic disease management, a lack of knowledge of allergies, medications, and relevant past medical histories of the residents. These issues then resulted in leading to significant adverse patient events.
5. In view of the rapid changeover of staff and the lack of involvement of the primary caregivers, there was inefficient clinical handover with respect to each resident. This resulted in adverse incidents to residents and also impacted the triaging of the residents in preparation for evacuation, as this was performed in the absence of relevant medical history.
6. There was a lack of command, control, and collaboration between all agencies involved in the evacuation, with unclear governance and a lack of clarity regarding roles, responsibilities, and accountability. This led to confusion, delays, and contributed to the adverse events experienced by the residents.

Key Lessons

1. Robust clinical governance policies and procedures need to be available, up-to-date, and regularly reviewed by all care providers who are trained and aware of their existence. This ensures that in an emergency all involved can expect to be well prepared and to prevent avoidable harm.
2. Clinical aspects of care, such as end-of-life care, medications prescribed, past medical history, and other relevant information, should be easily available in client records, regularly reviewed, and updated. This information should be part of the clinical handover and will assist in avoiding harm.
3. With the expansion of virtual care, telehealth, and other modes of clinical interaction, primary care providers can and should remain involved, even if 'off-site', e.g. in isolation or in their clinics. This would've significantly contributed to the care of the residents, avoided harm, and aided in the continuity of care.

16.5 Virtual Care Settings

The rapid expansion of virtual care, fuelled by technological advancements and evolving patient expectations, necessitates a robust framework for clinical governance. Such a framework ensures the provision of safe, effective, and high-quality care within the unique context of digital health delivery. Unlike traditional healthcare environments, virtual care presents distinct governance complexities relating to accessibility, data security, digital literacy, and the very nature of the patient-provider interaction.

Effective clinical governance in virtual care rests on a foundation of several core principles, mirroring those in traditional healthcare but requiring specific adaptation to the digital context. Appropriate policies and procedures will ensure that virtual care treatments are evidence based. Key to this is establishing patient admission criteria, modes of treatment delivery, the escalation of clinical deterioration, providing immediate support to clinicians managing patients virtually and managing the risks of diagnosing and treating by remote means. Successful virtual care services require involvement and engagement of the patient to ensure they have adequate digital technology at hand and they are adept at using such technologies, particularly when the patient is unwell.

Clinicians working in the virtual setting need education and training in the specific challenges that come with working in a remote environment. Additional privacy and data security measures are required in view of the reliance on technology from both the clinician and the patient. In the event of a clinical incident or poor clinical outcome, a robust process for reporting and managing adverse events and complaints in the remote environment is required. When implementing a virtual service, healthcare leaders need to ensure important clinical governance components are incorporated as part of normal service delivery.

Working with digital technology experts, the healthcare leader needs to ensure the appropriate selection of virtual platforms that are durable in terms of ongoing connectivity, privacy, security, and interoperability and interaction between clinicians and patients. Integration of this technology with an Electronic Medical Record (EMR) is key in the selection process. The virtual platform with an integrated EMR provides an opportunity for improved data collection, monitoring, and analysis, including patient-reported outcome and experience measures and adverse events. This requires integration with the organisation's incident management system, diagnostic-related coding software and clinical outcome and indicator databases.

Virtual care settings need to abide by the organisation's processes for monitoring and measuring clinical effectiveness, clinical review, and performance improvement. Clinicians working in the virtual space should have specific credentialing and scope of practice delineations and additional training and education to ensure they can practice safely in this challenging setting. Nevertheless, there continues to be significant challenges for healthcare leaders in ensuring the safety and quality of services delivered in virtual settings.

The rapid evolution of digital technology has the risk of placing significant pressure on the capacity of the organisation's clinical governance framework to keep pace. Whilst the adoption of virtual care settings by healthcare organisations to ease pressure on patient flow and occupancy within the walls of hospitals can bring clear advantages the issues of digital interoperability, risk of disconnect between patient and clinician, and growing regulatory compliance requirements may hamper their success.

Healthcare leaders should stay abreast of these difficulties and the rapid evolution of information in this space. Clinical governance is paramount to ensuring the safe, effective, and ethical delivery of virtual care services. By adopting a proactive, adaptable, and patient-centred approach, healthcare organisations can effectively navigate the complexities of this rapidly evolving field and fully leverage the potential of virtual care to improve health outcomes of patients. The integration of digital technologies with a strong foundation of clinical governance is therefore fundamental to the future of healthcare delivery.

17 Managing Impaired Clinicians

Managing impaired clinicians requires a structured and sensitive approach. Early identification, often through observable behavioural changes or performance discrepancies, is crucial.

A clear, confidential reporting mechanism must be in place which adheres to relevant legal and ethical guidelines. Once identified, a thorough assessment by qualified professionals, often involving addiction specialists or mental health experts, is necessary to determine the extent of the impairment. Rehabilitation and monitoring programs, tailored to the clinician's specific needs, should be considered and established where relevant. Return-to-work protocols must be carefully defined, emphasising patient safety and ongoing oversight. The focus should be on both supporting the clinician's recovery and ensuring the highest standards of professional practice.

Clinician practitioners are regulated by various boards and licensing agencies. In this section, the Australian regulatory system will be used to discuss the key issues relating to managing clinician impairment. In Australia, clinician practitioners are required to be registered with the Australian Health Practitioner Regulation Agency (AHPRA) to clinically practice under the Health Practitioner Regulation National Law Act (National Law).

Under the National Law, as it's in force in each state and territory, clinician impairment is one of the grounds for both voluntary and mandatory notifications that must be made to the Medical Board of Australia under specific circumstances.

17.1 What Is Clinician Impairment?

The National Law defines clinician impairment as:

A physical or mental impairment, disability, condition or disorder (including substance abuse or dependence) that detrimentally affects or is likely to detrimentally affect:

© The Author(s), under exclusive license to Springer Nature Singapore Pte Ltd. 2026
L. Prado, S. Chandrasiri, *The Practice of Clinical Governance*, https://doi.org/10.1007/978-981-19-7896-8_17

(a) *for a registered health practitioner or an applicant for registration in a health profession, the person's capacity to practise the profession; or*
(b) *for a student, the student's capacity to undertake clinical training as part of the approved program of study in which the student is enrolled or as arranged by an education provider.*

Anyone can make a notification about a medical practitioner who they believe may be impaired.

The 'National Law' provides protection from civil, criminal, and administrative liability for persons who make a notification in good faith.

17.1.1 Grounds for Voluntary Notifications Related to Impairment

A voluntary notification can be made if:

A practitioner has, or may have, an impairment.
A practitioner has, or may have, contravened a condition on their registration or an undertaking given to the Board.

17.1.2 Grounds for Mandatory Notifications Related to Impairment

Grounds for mandatory notifications include impairment in relation to 'notifiable conduct'.

With respect to registered medical practitioners with an impairment, notifiable conduct includes circumstances where the practitioner has:

Practised their profession while intoxicated by alcohol or drugs.
Placed the public at risk of substantial harm because the practitioner's practice has been impacted by an impairment.

17.1.3 Actions the Board Can Take After Assessment of an Impaired Practitioner Notification

The Medical Board has the power to take a range of actions at any time after a health assessment.

These actions include:

A decision to take no further action.
Referral to another entity, such as a health complaints entity or
Immediate action if this is necessary to protect the health and safety of the public.

Issue a caution to the medical practitioner and/or
Require acceptance of an undertaking from them and/or
Impose conditions on the practitioner's registration.

17.2 The Role of the Healthcare Leader in Managing Impaired Clinicians

As leaders with accountability for clinical governance of healthcare organisations, there are two key components of the clinical governance framework that directly relate to the responsibility for managing impaired clinicians. These include maintaining an 'effective clinical workforce' and ensuring appropriate 'risk management'.

In order to maintain an effective clinical workforce whilst balancing the risk of any impairment, health leaders need to ensure the clinicians within their organisation are able to fulfil their professional and personal responsibilities for patient care. Current estimates suggest that approximately up to 15% of physicians will be impaired at some point in their careers (Boisaubin and Levine 2001). Common causes include impairment due to psychiatric illness and/or alcohol and/or drug dependency. There are many background factors that could predispose medical practitioners to an impairment, including personality factors such as the drive for improvement, ambition, and conscientiousness.

With respect to clinicians, there is often a high likelihood of denying any personal problems. Identifying impairment, if mild or in the initial stages of manifestation, is therefore often difficult. It is critical that health leaders are trained and knowledgeable in identifying such impairment early since patient safety is at stake, and if untreated, impairment may lead to catastrophic implications for the clinician themselves, including loss of registration, and health issues, including mental health disorders. Death by suicide is unfortunately higher in the health professions.

17.3 Practical Approach to the Management of an Impaired Clinician

The key overarching concerns for a health leader when faced with a potentially impaired practitioner include:

1. Ensuring the safety of patients.
2. Ensuring the safety and appropriate management of the practitioner.
3. Minimising any adverse impact on the immediate surroundings, such as other staff and potential adverse impact on clinical operations.
4. Managing self and complying with reporting obligations.

When an allegation or potential concern relating to medical practitioner impairment is raised, the health leader must assess any impact on the safety of any current patients and/or staff, whilst working to verify the accuracy of any allegations. This should occur simultaneously, however, safety precautions are often required and advisable to be enacted on the premise that such allegations may be true. This will include consideration of the clinical impact on any current inpatients or outpatients of the medical practitioner, any patients that are booked to be seen by the practitioner in the immediate future, and any who may have been treated in the past.

An immediate and urgent meeting, or at the very least a phone call with the practitioner is recommended to gauge the level and extent of intervention that is required. This may result in arrangements requiring the transfer of patients for care or follow-up to another practitioner, rescheduling of appointments/theatre cases, and/or ensuring a chaperon/proctor is allocated to assist/temporarily work with the impacted practitioner.

The immediate safety of the practitioner themselves warrants cautious and immediate action. This may include engaging the services of police, acute mental health services and/or family members, particularly when there may be concerns regarding the acute risk of suicide or drug and alcohol abuse. The practitioner may be required to be temporarily suspended from practice and/or removed from the environment for a period of time. It is advisable to take all such immediate actions with the mutual agreement and discussion with the practitioner wherever possible.

In each case it is essential to consider and manage the risk to patient safety, whilst also safeguarding the reputational risk to both the clinician themselves and the health service. In addition, it is important to consider any potential immediate adverse impact to staff and colleagues of the clinician. It is prudent to undertake such actions under strict and appropriate privacy and confidentiality measures.

In the event that it may be difficult for a health leader to accurately gauge the clinical impact or risk of an impaired practitioner's conduct in order to action any immediate safeguards, the enlisting of expert clinical opinion from an appropriate senior specialist of the same practising specialty as the clinician is recommended. This may be the clinical director of the department, head of unit, an internal or external senior specialist, and/or the relevant speciality college.

Appropriate communication in relation to any immediate restrictions that are placed or immediate interventions undertaken will be required to be shared with all relevant stakeholders on a 'need to know basis', whilst maintaining the privacy and confidentiality of the clinician as much as possible. This may include the need to escalate and inform the CEO, Board, and/or other external governance and/or regulatory bodies. Some of these reporting requirements may be mandated and stated in applicable legislation.

The timing, format, and tone of the formal meeting with the impaired practitioner requires a considered approach and is dependent on the findings from the initial meeting with the clinician and the preliminary gathering of facts. The immediate and urgent meeting to verify and come to an agreement on acute interventions or actions should be done face to face whenever possible, however it may be quite appropriate under certain circumstances to be done via a phone call. The more formal and structured meetings for further exploration, discussion, and/or decision-making can occur in a less urgent timeframe.

It may be relevant for the health leader to obtain comprehensive information on a range of performance and conduct measures involving the clinician before a structured and formal meeting, in order to better understand the degree of impairment and plan for remediation or other actions into the longer term.

17.3.1 Internal Review of Impaired Practitioner

A comprehensive review of the performance and conduct of the concerned practitioner often involves discussions with his/her colleagues and other staff, particularly relating to patterns of behaviour. Further aspects in the preliminary/internal review include the following:

(a) *Formal or informal complaints* against the practitioner. These may be accessed via the hospital's incident management system, confidential files in workforce units, and/or HR departments. It should involve a collation and review of any complaints made by staff, patients, students, and/or colleagues. The process used to resolve and manage those complaints should also be assessed, and any patterns in the nature and trend of complaints should also be taken into consideration.

(b) *Credentialing status including the scope of clinical practice.* The relevant 'Board' registration status, noting any recent conditions or restrictions, and the credentialing status of the practitioner warrants review. This includes a detailed assessment of the scope of clinical practice that the practitioner holds at the health service and/or other health services. It must be cross-referenced against his/her clinical activity to verify that the clinician has been/is practising within his/her scope. This is particularly relevant in the context of surgical procedures, and all activity performed by the clinician can be obtained from the health information services of the organisation e.g. via coded data. Clinical audits, peer review reports, and mortality and morbidity reviews may be further sources for identifying whether any concerns regarding their practice exist, including identifying any cases that were outside the practitioner's clinical scope.

(c) *Activity levels*: Activity and procedure volumes and types should be compared against the practitioner's peers and within the organisation. The frequency, volume, and types of procedures performed should be comparable to those with similar experience and qualifications and should align with the clinical capability of the health service. Health organisations may have clinical activity dashboards that can be utilised for this, or health information services, audits, and case review activities are often also appropriate sources for these.

    Concerns regarding competency may arise if the practitioner's activity levels of a certain procedure or at a particular site within the health service are found to be too low. This raises issues of the clinician's familiarity with the team and the hospital's clinical protocols, as well as their level of competence, which is normally strengthened through adequate exposure and experience in doing a particular procedure frequently.

(d) *Clinical outcomes and operational measures*: Reviewing the data provided to or obtained from internal and external registries, coding data, and incident management systems is important to undertake. Assessing clinical outcomes, including mortality rates, hospital-acquired complication rates, post-operative complications such as perforations, anastomosis leaks, and surgical site infections, and common reasons for prolonged ICU stays or reasons for unplanned readmissions, and benchmarking these with the rates of his/her peers will provide a good understanding of the practitioner's level of performance.

Operational measures such as the lengths of stay, unplanned returns to theatre rates, readmission rates, procedure durations, and admission and discharge patterns of his/her patients will help to identify any clinical practice outliers or significant deviations from peer-accepted guidelines.

17.3.2 Meeting with the Impaired Practitioner

Once the health leader has a good understanding of the practitioner's past and recent overall practice, outcomes, conduct, and behaviour, a formal meeting may be organised to discuss the concerns relating to any impaired practice.

Ensuring procedural fairness and affording natural justice for the medical practitioner throughout the investigation and management of impaired practice or conduct is of the utmost importance. This includes enabling their right to reply to any allegations made, the right to be fully informed of any allegations made, the right to an appropriate period of notice of any meetings that are planned, and their right to have appropriate professional and/or personal support available at any meetings or discussions.

Minimising any actual or perceived bias and conflicts of interest when organising and conducting such meetings, particularly regarding who is involved in such meetings or deliberations, is critical. Conducting the meetings and undertaking any communications with the impaired practitioner must be done with a high degree of sensitivity and support and in a manner that safeguards their right to privacy and confidentiality.

A letter to be issued outlining the allegations, initial findings, and a formal request for a meeting with adequate notice is good practice. This should also formally state their right to bring with them a support person and the means of providing access to any medical files or hospital systems that they may require in order to prepare their response ahead of any formal meetings.

It is advisable to prepare and plan for the meeting, including assessing the set-up of the meeting room, with consideration being given to aspects such as safety and alarm systems should they be required by the health leader at any point during the meeting and any backup support, such as security, that may need to be on standby should it be required. Meeting the clinician accompanied by another member of the leadership team, such as a head of unit or a legal or human resources representative, can also be considered, however, care must be taken to ensure that meetings are conducted in environments and circumstances that are perceived by the clinician as non-threatening.

The format of the meeting will usually involve an explanation of the concerns or findings followed by adequate time given to actively listen to the response by the clinician. During this interaction, the health leader can make a professional assessment of the clinician's physical and psychological state, including an assessment of the level of risk that may be posed to themselves and/or others.

Means of resolving issues or access to intervention and treatment can be discussed, including any requirements to undertake mandatory reporting to regulatory agencies. Expectations regarding future behaviour, supervision requirements, or monitoring arrangements (e.g. for alcohol/drug testing), or any restrictions on their existing scope of clinical practice can be discussed with the clinician and their support person, with clear agreement reached as to the next steps.

During this discussion, the health leader must make an assessment of the clinician's:

1. Capacity for insight: whether the clinician understands and accepts the level of impairment that may exist.
2. Capacity for reflection: whether the clinician can reflect on and understand how others may have been/could be affected or impacted by their impaired practice.
3. Capacity for judgement: whether the clinician can formulate a rational approach to remediate or resolve or get assistance to address any impairment.
4. Commitment and preparedness to change and improve.

This approach to assessment will assist greatly in reaching the necessary level of response that is required in each instance.

The art of managing the impaired practitioner in an effective, sensitive, and appropriate way requires a mature and empathic approach to be utilised by the health leader. Balancing the need for privacy and confidentiality for the clinician with the requirement for open disclosure and obligatory reporting, whilst affording the clinician procedural fairness and natural justice at all times is needed. Communicating appropriately to then reach mutually agreed decisions where possible, whilst safeguarding the safety and reputation of all involved, is what will determine the difference between successful or unsuccessful management of these complex situations.

17.4 Case Study 1: Impaired Doctor

The safety and quality officer receives a complaint from the operating theatre technician claiming that an anaesthetist has been leaving cases mid-operation, for up to 15 min at a time, on a regular basis to 'go on toilet breaks' over the last few weeks. The staff are concerned because the doctor appears disoriented and vague at times following these breaks.

Whilst there have been no clinical incidents to note, there have been a few 'minor issues' with failure to follow policies, which have been attributed to 'fatigue', 'work pressure', and 'forgetfulness'. The anaesthetist is well considered and liked by the team and her colleagues. There have been no concerns regarding her clinical performance, and generally, there are no incidents concerning the diversion of drugs from the theatre complex.

The safety and quality officer has raised the issue with the Head of Unit. The Head of Unit had spoken with the doctor, who was apparently agitated in response, stating she was feeling victimised by staff for 'reporting her'. She had explained that the absences related to a medical condition. She had been angry and aggressive during this encounter and has demanded an apology. As a consequence, there had been no further actions taken.

Two weeks later, the doctor collapses whilst operating in the theatre shortly after returning from the bathroom. A medical emergency code is called, and the doctor is clinically reviewed. Upon recovering, she reassures the medical team that she had just fainted and that there are no concerns regarding her health. The Chief Medical Officer is now informed.

The CMO meets with the Head of Unit, who is very concerned. She states that the anaesthetist's behaviour from a social perspective has noticeably changed over the last few months. She had become increasingly withdrawn, avoided social interaction with the group, and missed a number of clinical meetings. The Head of Unit is concerned her colleague may be depressed, as her mood seems to have remained flat and her affect blunted. It is noted that she had been through a recent relationship breakup and had also recently volunteered for additional after-hours shifts.

The CMO decides to meet with the anaesthetist. Initially, at the meeting, the doctor appears agitated, and her mood swings from passive-aggressive to apologetic and contrite over a short period of time. The CMO explains to her that her recent 'collapse' has meant that colleagues are concerned to work with her. The doctor discloses that she is yet to undertake the clinical investigations after her 'faint' and follow-up review that had been suggested to her by the medical team.

The CMO discusses with her his concerns particularly regarding her recent:

- Behaviour, both in the theatre and in these discussions.
- Recent collapse at work.
- Failure to undertake the clinical reviews.
- Recent stressors, concerns, and problems.

The CMO asks her:

- If she has a regular primary care physician.
- If she has had any recent medical issues, which she should disclose.
- Current alcohol and drug use, including any 'illicit' agents.
- About her mood, memory, concentration, and other mental health questions, including any suicidal ideation.

From her responses, the CMO is concerned that the doctor is currently not fit for work and requests that:

- She goes on sick leave.
- Attends her primary care physician.
- Obtains medical clearance before returning to work.

The anaesthetist takes 2 weeks of sick leave and returns with a clearance from her physician. Her behaviour seems improved and remains so over the next 3 months. She is then found one day unconscious in the theatre bathroom.

A detailed review is undertaken, led by the CMO, which identifies that the doctor is regularly using drugs at work.

Consequently, the CMO arranges for:

- Immediate medical assistance for the doctor, who is argumentative, to enter a rehabilitation facility, where both her drug and mental health issues can be addressed.
- Notification to the medical regulatory board.
- Review of the doctor's clinical care over the last 2 years.
- A meeting with the Head of Unit to ensure confidentiality and arrange appropriate clinical cover.

Over the next months, the doctor is enrolled in a Medical Board-approved drug and alcohol rehabilitation program and a return-to-work plan, which includes:

- Ongoing drug testing.
- Ongoing mental health sessions.
- Allocation of a supervisor/mentor.
- Regular clinical review sessions with an allocated senior specialist.
- Regular meetings with the CMO.

Over the following 18 months, the doctor's performance remains stable and satisfactory. Her mood seems to improve, although her social interactions remain minimal. The CMO is then advised that she has not attended work for 2 days and is uncontactable. A welfare check is subsequently arranged, and she is found to have died at her home by completed suicide. The department, hospital staff, and the CMO are extremely impacted by this news.

Management of the impaired medical practitioner is a difficult scenario for healthcare leaders. Despite best efforts, particularly when the dual diagnosis of alcohol and drug use exists, the outcomes in such cases are difficult to predict.

Therefore, healthcare leaders need to have a focus on clinician wellbeing, including 'burnout', to help prevent harm to doctors as early as possible and to help ensure the continued wellbeing of the workforce.

Important features of such a clinician well-being program include the following:

- Comprehensive clinician well-being strategies with a focus on education and training on aspects of 'self-care'.
- Training for leaders to recognise and identify signs of deteriorating mental health status, and how to ask colleagues about their wellbeing.
- Access to primary care, physicians, and specialists in addiction medicine, mental health, and appropriate psychological and social wellbeing services.
- Mentorship/peer support programs.
- Early detection of an impaired clinician using a number of 'red flag' identifiers such as:
  - Attendance, mood, and tone.
  - Social interactions and avoidance behaviour.
  - Clinical performance and outcomes.
  - Unusual practices or behaviour.
  - Complaints and concerns raised.

Access to rehabilitation programs and return-to-work programs, including adequate monitoring, peer supports, and independent reviews that meet jurisdictional requirements is critical in the management of impaired clinicians.

Further Reading

Medical Board of Australia. Information on the management of impaired practitioners. 20 January 2012.

Boisaubin EV, Levine RE. Identifying and assisting the impaired physician. Am J Med Sci. 2001 Jul;322(1):31–6. https://doi.org/10.1097/00000441-200107000-00006.

GPSR Compliance

The European Union's (EU) General Product Safety Regulation (GPSR) is a set of rules that requires consumer products to be safe and our obligations to ensure this.

If you have any concerns about our products, you can contact us on ProductSafety@springernature.com

In case Publisher is established outside the EU, the EU authorized representative is:

Springer Nature Customer Service Center GmbH
Europaplatz 3
69115 Heidelberg, Germany

Batch number: 10351347

Printed by Printforce, the Netherlands